D1297976

The
World According to
TODDLERS

Other books by
Shannon Payette Seip and Adrienne Hedger

• •

If These Boobs Could Talk
Momnesia

The World According to TODDLERS

Shannon Payette Seip and Adrienne Hedger

Andrews McMeel Publishing, LLC

Kansas City · Sydney · London

The World According to Toddlers

Copyright © 2011 by Shannon Payette Seip and Adrienne Hedger. Illustrations copyright © 2011 by Adrienne Hedger. All rights reserved. Printed in China. No part of this book may be used or reproduced in any manner whatsoever without written permission except in the case of reprints in the context of reviews. For information, write Andrews McMeel Publishing, LLC, an Andrews McMeel Universal company, 1130 Walnut Street, Kansas City, Missouri 64106.

11 12 13 14 15 WKT 10 9 8 7 6 5 4 3 2 1

ISBN: 978-1-4494-0120-7

Library of Congress Control Number: 2010930543

www.andrewsmcmeel.com

Book design by Diane Marsh

Cover design by Julie Barnes

ATTENTION: SCHOOLS AND BUSINESSES
Andrews McMeel books are available at quantity discounts with bulk purchase for educational, business, or sales promotional use. For information, please write to: Special Sales Department, Andrews McMeel Publishing, LLC, 1130 Walnut Street, Kansas City, Missouri 64106.

CONTENTS

Introduction vii

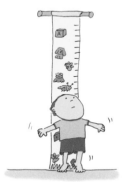

Chapter 1
Major Milestones 1

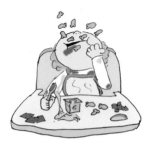

Chapter 2
Munch Time! 21

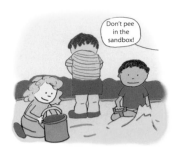

Chapter 3
The Social Lives of Toddlers 41

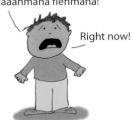

Chapter 4
Use Your Words 61

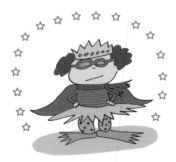

Chapter 5
Grooming 77

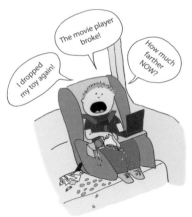

Chapter 6
On the Go! 93

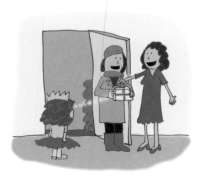

Chapter 7
Where's My Present? 107

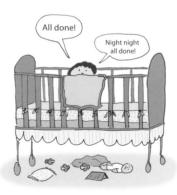

Chapter 8
Night-Night! 125

INTRODUCTION

In the beginning they are babies. Cue the soft music... ♫ ♪ 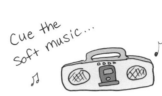 ♪ Lullaby and goodnight

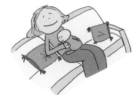

So cuddly. So sweet.

Eating enthusiastically.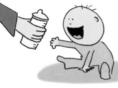

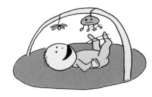

Playing happily.

Wearing the outfits you choose.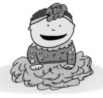

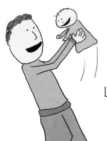

Life is good.

Then, around 18 months, the world starts to change.

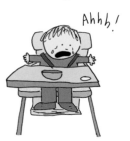

One day, out of nowhere, they *do not* want to be strapped into their high chair.

They develop shockingly strong opinions about toys.

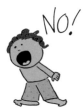

And there is *no way* they are wearing that shirt you picked out.

This is when you realize: Your baby is gone . . . and in its place is a boisterous, opinionated, and amazingly imaginative human: your toddler.

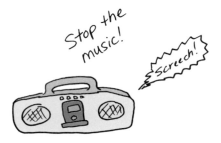

Welcome to the World According to Toddlers—a hilarious, messy, and unpredictable universe.

In this world, you will face absurd demands, exasperating behavior, and crazy displays of willpower and negotiation. But you'll also experience adorable, heartwarming moments—moments that will remind you why you are doing all this.

The best way to navigate the toddler world: *appreciate the humor.* After all, when else will you live with someone who firmly believes he is the boss of you but only comes up to your knee? When else will you get a glimpse into a fascinating world where food must be cut *just* so? A world where there is only *one* acceptable outfit and it must be worn over and over? A world where throwing a spectacular tantrum is a daily action item?

Let's take a look at the World According to Toddlers, in all its glory and absurdity. And let's find the humor so we can appreciate these miniature people before they outgrow this once-in-a-lifetime stage.

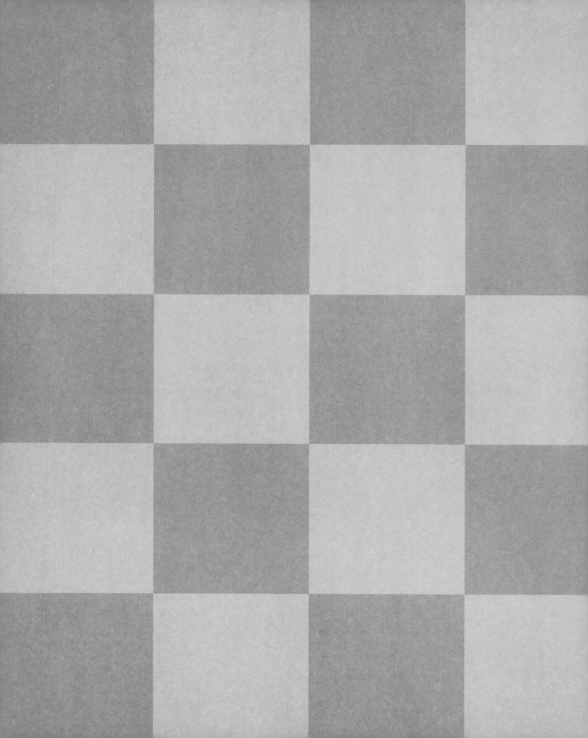

Chapter 1

Major MILESTONES

a.k.a. What You're in For

So you have yourself a toddler—a tiny little munchkin who tries to run the show. At first this new behavior is pretty adorable: The way he crosses his arms. The way she says "No!" so emphatically.

Then . . . less cute. And you start to wonder: "What am I in for here? Where is all this headed?"

Here are some of the key behaviors and milestones that mark the growth and development of toddlers—the good, the bad, and the utterly ridiculous.

SET YOUR EXPECTATIONS

To successfully coexist with toddlers, you need to have the right expectations. Here's what the experts say—and what it means for you.

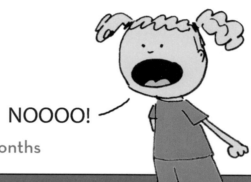

NOOOO!

Between 12 and 18 months

Experts Say Toddler Should Be Able To . . .	What This Means for You
Use one to fifteen words	At first, great excitement and delight. My baby can talk! Then, a seed of doubt. Was it possibly better back in the days when he *couldn't* talk?
Play by throwing objects and picking them up	Don't count on the "picking up" part.
Walk well alone; creep up stairs	You will be yelling, "Ack! Where did you go?!" a lot.

Between 18 and 24 months

Experts Say Toddler Should Be Able To . . .	What This Means for You
Run well	Ready for a workout?
Fall easily	Toddler's obsession with Band-Aids begins.
Continue practicing using the spoon	Your patience will be tested to the extreme as you watch yet another stack of peas roll off the spoon and onto the tray and floor. Secretly, you fear your kid will *never* master the spoon. Never!

At age 2

Experts Say Toddler Should Be Able To . . .	What This Means for You
Take off an article of clothing	Get ready to see a nude toddler at every turn.
Entertain an imaginary friend	This imaginary friend will want a real cookie. And she will order the toddler to eat the cookie.
Draw a vertical line	. . . on the tile floor, wall, or couch—in permanent marker.

At age 3

Experts Say Toddler Should Be Able To . . .	What This Means for You
Put together a six-piece puzzle	. . . then promptly lose two pieces forever.
Ask who, what, where, and why questions	. . . over and over and over and over and over.
Solve problems if they are simple, concrete, real, and immediate	Such as: How can I cover my whole body with this protein powder I just found in the pantry?

IMPRESSIVE . . . RIGHT?

These seem like great achievements—until you look at other animals and what they can accomplish. For example, the giraffe.

Giraffe Milestones

- On their feet within twenty minutes of being born
- Run within twenty-four hours of birth
- Become fully independent by fifteen months

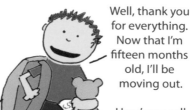

Well, thank you for everything. Now that I'm fifteen months old, I'll be moving out.

Here's my cell number. Keep in touch.

TEN LIKELY CAUSES OF TANTRUMS

1. You picked out a shirt with buttons.

2. You won't let Toddler wear one shamrock sock and nothing else.

3. You put a purple lid on the orange sippy cup.

4. You pushed the garage door opener instead of letting Toddler push it.

5. You put Toddler in car seat.

6. You tried to take Toddler out of car seat.

7. You mentioned the words "car seat."

8. Sibling looked at Toddler's toy.

9. You did not let Toddler buy sixty-ounce bag of marshmallows.

10. You wouldn't tuck Toddler in for tenth time.

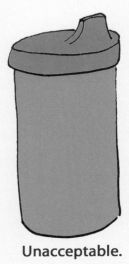

Unacceptable.

T A N T R U M
B I N G O

Which behaviors are you seeing today?

Launches into tantrum without warning	Screams for eighteen seconds without taking breath	Throws self on floor	Chucks object at your head	Tries to chuck another object but accidentally hits self with it
Gets up and throws self on floor again	Silent screams (mouth open, no sound) for more than ten seconds	Spits	Appears to be break dancing, except for the sobbing	Pees on floor to spite you
Bites corner of wall	Inadvertently performs a beautiful scissor-kick	Staggers around, following you wherever you go	Growls like Mufasa from *The Lion King*	Yanks all clothes out of drawers
Crowd of twelve people watching	Shopping cart involved	Refuses to let go of candy	Removes shoe and throws it at wall	Wants shoe back and becomes even more outraged
Passionately shouts words no one can understand	Face turns color of eggplant	Bangs forehead against hard object	Smacks pacifier away when offered	Falls asleep from exhaustion

THE UPSIDE

Tantrum again? Look at the bright side: Since ignoring it is really your only option, you finally have a moment to get something done.

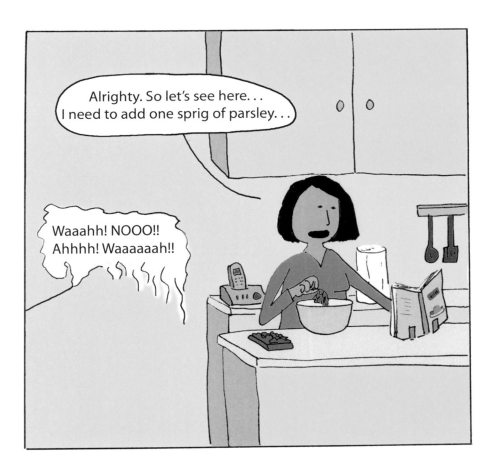

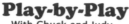

Play-by-Play
With Chuck and Judy

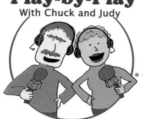

A MAJOR UPSET

A tantrum is brewing. Let's cut to our commentators, Chuck and Judy, who are live on the scene to give us a play-by-play report.

Chuck, I sense Toddler is growing dissatisfied.

Well, look at those shoes Mom is asking her to wear. Tennis shoes with Velcro? That's outrageous! Why can't Toddler wear those fancy shoes?

I think we're about to witness a full-blown tantrum. Let's watch the technique.

Toddler is growing more irate. . . . Judy, the crying has commenced.

She's yelling something. . . . I can't quite make it out.

Well, we can hear the word "no" for sure.

She's making a move to throw herself to the ground. Wait . . . she's holding back on the sobbing while she concentrates on lowering herself to the ground . . . carefully.

The sobbing resumes, Judy!

Even more powerful than before.

Watch that arm and leg movement. Impressive.
Now she's rolling onto her stomach.

Chuck, the rear end is lifting into the air, and now
Toddler is banging her forehead on the ground. Ouch!

Wait, now she's rolling to her back again. . . .
She's kicking wildly at the air.

Chuck, everything is infuriating to her now. Even air.

She's punching the air! I would not want to be
that air right now. And listen to that scream!

This kid knows her stuff.

Well, she's had practice, Judy. Plenty of practice.

Next: Chuck and Judy visit a toddler at snack time.

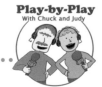

Play-by-Play
With Chuck and Judy

PACIFIER: TIME TO SAY GOOD-BYE?

Is today the day that Toddler should give up the pacifier forever? And are you ready to fight this battle? Use this handy chart to find out.

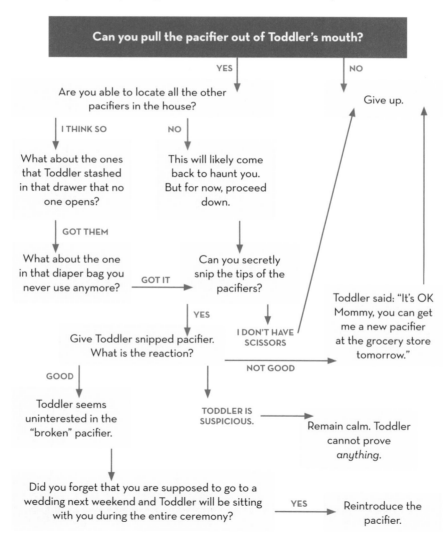

Can you pull the pacifier out of Toddler's mouth?

YES

NO

Are you able to locate all the other pacifiers in the house?

Give up.

I THINK SO

NO

What about the ones that Toddler stashed in that drawer that no one opens?

This will likely come back to haunt you. But for now, proceed down.

GOT THEM

What about the one in that diaper bag you never use anymore?

GOT IT

Can you secretly snip the tips of the pacifiers?

Toddler said: "It's OK Mommy, you can get me a new pacifier at the grocery store tomorrow."

YES

Give Toddler snipped pacifier. What is the reaction?

I DON'T HAVE SCISSORS

NOT GOOD

GOOD

Toddler seems uninterested in the "broken" pacifier.

TODDLER IS SUSPICIOUS.

Remain calm. Toddler cannot prove *anything*.

Did you forget that you are supposed to go to a wedding next weekend and Toddler will be sitting with you during the entire ceremony?

YES

Reintroduce the pacifier.

Eulogy to a Pacifier

When the time comes to retire the pacifier, it's only fitting to hold a memorial service for this precious piece of plastic. Here's a guide if you're at a loss for words:

Dear _____ (Pacifier, Passy, Binky, Fussplug, etc.),

Your time with us was so short, and yet about eight months too long.

You were the only thing that made Toddler calm down and regain his sanity. I'd like to say that there's no one like you, but truth be told, there are millions just like you, each for $2.49 on aisle 7B.

You never got mad when Toddler dropped you on the ground and didn't bother to wash you off before popping you back in. And you showed stoic courage that time you were trapped under the car seat for weeks, gathering lint and slowly becoming deformed.

You never minded the glares from strangers who seemed to think you didn't belong anymore. They had no idea that if it weren't for you, Toddler would have transformed into the Tasmanian Devil.

I would ask that we have a moment of silence to remember you, but ironically this is not possible because we need you to induce the silence. So instead we'll have a moment of loud crying. I might be crying the loudest.

You Are My Stuffed Toy

An ode to stuffed animals, sung to the tune of "You Are My Sunshine."

You are my stuffed toy,
One of a hundred,
And I am poking your eyeballs out.
I'm using marker
To make you purple
And I'm blowing my nose on your face.

You are my stuffed toy,
My little stuffed toy,
And I am dragging you through the dirt.
Now I am sucking
On your left ear
And putting three diapers on you.

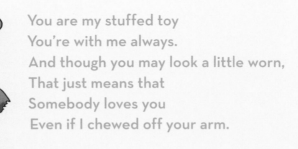

You are my stuffed toy
You're with me always.
And though you may look a little worn,
That just means that
Somebody loves you
Even if I chewed off your arm.

The Old Switcheroo

Did you accidentally lose your toddler's favorite blankie and try to replace it with what you considered an identical blankie? Nice try. In the World of Toddlers, there are *no substitutions*.

How *you* see the situation:

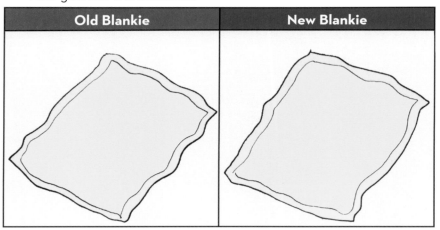

How your *toddler* sees the situation:

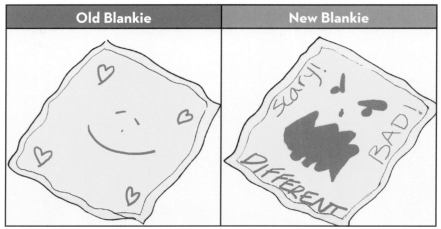

Toddler Handbook

TIPS FOR TODDLERS, BY TODDLERS

POTTY-TRAINING BASICS

- It's best to remove all your clothing before you use the toilet.

- Wiping is optional. Always.

- The ideal times to go to the bathroom are when you and your mom are in a pool; in the car during a traffic jam; when you are about to check out at the grocery store; when you finally get to the front of a very, very long line at an amusement park.

- You and only you must flush the toilet. No exceptions. Ever.

- Beware of public toilets. They will suck you down with the flush.

Note: If you are not ready to poop on the toilet, just poop in your pull-up. Do not announce your intentions to anyone; instead, hide in a corner or crouch behind something, then go to work. If your mom sees you she will just think, "Oh, he is hiding and has a very serious look on his face." *She will not guess what you are actually doing.*

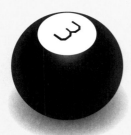

Ask the Magic 3 Ball

Ask the Magic 3 Ball and tap into a three-year-old's wisdom

Toddler: Will I get rewarded with "potty-training" jelly beans if I play with Mommy's hairbrush in the potty?

Magic 3 Ball:

Certainly not.

But you will get a dramatic reaction if you show her how you can brush your teeth with your newfound bigger "toothbrush."

TODDLER HANDBOOK
TIPS FOR TODDLERS, BY TODDLERS

BATHROOM "TOP FIVE" LISTS
Top Five Best Uses for a Portable Toilet

- Drum
- Storage for toys
- Science experiment: How much water can be poured in until it overflows?
- Helmet when riding tricycle
- Piggy bank

Top Five Things to Do in a Public Restroom

- Touch the toilet after your mom says don't.
- Wash your hands, then touch the floor.
- Insist on dispensing the soap and paper towels all by yourself, even if you can't reach.
- Keep activating the automatic paper towel dispenser.
- Overreact to the noise of the loud hand dryer.

How to Do the Potty Dance

✐ In answer to your mother's question, tell her, "No, I NO gotta go potty."

✐ Insist that you do not even need to try.

✐ Five minutes after you leave the bathroom vicinity, start the dance.

✐ Cross and bend legs.

✐ Arrange face into a grimace.

✐ Bounce rapidly.

✐ Jump from foot to foot.

✐ Sway your shoulders to and fro.

✐ Immediately sit criss-cross-applesauce wherever you are.

✐ Shriek, "Yes, gotta go potty! I gotta go now! It's coming out!"

✐ Enjoy the fun, bouncy ride you will receive after your mom scoops you up and runs with you back to the bathroom. Whee!

You Did It!

According to toddlers, going to the bathroom on the potty is a huge deal, no matter how old you are. So bask in the attention. You've earned it.

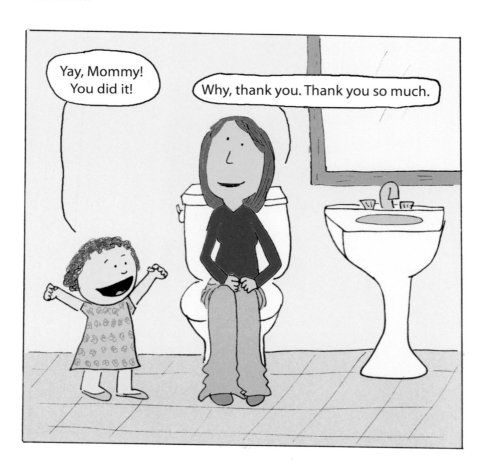

WHERE IT'S ALL HEADED

Do you observe Toddler's behavior and fear how it will shape the future? If Toddler can just channel it properly, the possibilities are limitless!

Toddler's Current Behavior	What You're Afraid Of	If It's Channeled Correctly
Nonstop lying	Becomes a con man	Becomes a top spy
Drama queen	Remains a drama queen	Becomes a soap opera star
Bossy	Becomes an angry, heartless drill sergeant	Becomes an incredible fitness instructor
Overly attached to one special blankie	Becomes an adult who is *still* overly attached to one special blankie	Becomes a very loyal spouse
Very picky eating	Constant threat of malnourishment	Becomes world renowned food critic for *The New York Times*

FLIP-FLOPPED

What would happen if adults behaved like toddlers?

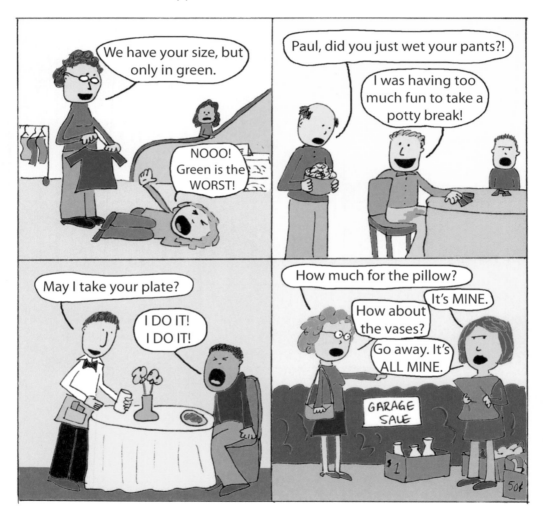

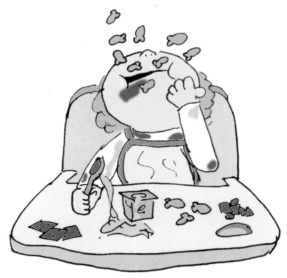

Chapter 2

MUNCH TIME!

A juice box chilled at exactly thirty-seven degrees. Hexagonal wheat crackers, arranged in a fan. Green grapes that are perfectly oblong.

No, it's not a superstar's dressing room requirements; it's the high-maintenance demands of a toddler.

When it comes to food that pleases your toddler, you may feel like a reality show contestant trying to please a finicky judge. (If you're so lucky as to have a kid who eats anything, feel free to skip this chapter knowing we are all envious of the sushi platter your family is sharing tonight.)

Napkins on laps! Let's dig into the world of toddlers and food.

TODDLER HANDBOOK
TIPS FOR TODDLERS, BY TODDLERS

PREPARING TO EAT

- Take newly washed hands and rub them on floor, bottom of shoe, or equally unsanitary surface.

- Strip down to nothing or demand to put on a brand-new white shirt.

- Mentally prepare for a plate full of fresh cookies. Resolve to accept nothing less.

- Let the meal begin.

THE TODDLER FOOD PYRAMID

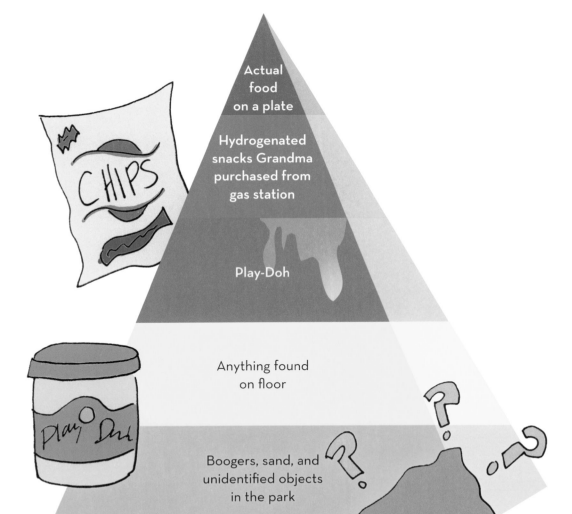

A FINE, FINE LINE

Food preparation is an area with no gray zones. The food is either served the *correct* way or the *infuriatingly incorrect* way. Let's take a look.

Edible

French toast cut into squares

Applesauce presented in a single-serve plastic container

Corn

A cracker

Banana that is *perfectly* yellow all over

Piece of cheese on someone else's plate

Obviously Inedible

French toast cut into rectangles

Applesauce dumped out of container and presented in a bowl

Corn that is touching the food next to it

A cracker that has a slight chip off the corner

Nearly perfect yellow banana with one tiny brown dot on the peel

Same piece of cheese on Toddler's plate

OPEN UP!

Some toddlers need a little extra incentive before they'll open up for a bite. Here are some strategies to consider. Start at the top and move down, depending on how desperate you become.

Optimistic

"Choo-choo! Open up, here comes the train!"

Forget the plate! Present the food in a different container; for example, an espresso cup or a Crock-Pot.

Douse it with condiments. Ketchup, ranch, sprinkles—whatever it takes. Mix them all together, if needed.

Arrange the condiment-smothered food into an intriguing sculpture. Think Eiffel Tower or Stonehenge.

Try to steal the masterpiece from your toddler. Shout "Mine!" and lunge for it.

Oh, forget it! Convince yourself that somehow mac and cheese four times a day will help your toddler grow into a fine, healthy person.

Desperate

INTRODUCING NEW FOOD?
GOOD LUCK WITH THAT

A typical toddler needs multiple exposures to a new food before he'll even *think* about tasting it. But what parent wants to keep making broccoli only to have it rejected twelve times? Instead of trying new recipes, try these strategies:

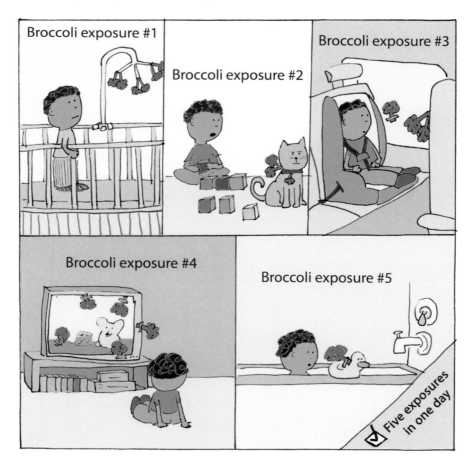

TODDLER HANDBOOK
TIPS FOR TODDLERS, BY TODDLERS

HOW TO USE A STRAW

- Admire straw.

- Bend straw.

- Flick straw out of drink. Spray droplets of beverage on self and those nearby.

- Look at your mother. What is she all upset over?! Sheesh.

- Put mouth on straw. Do not suck beverage into straw; instead, blow really hard and create bubbles until someone orders you to stop.

- With straw in mouth, tip cup toward you.

- Spill beverage all over clothing. Complain that straw is not working.

- Once you are in new clothes, repeat.

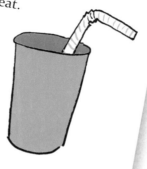

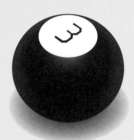

Ask the Magic 3 Ball

Ask the Magic 3 Ball and
tap into a three-year-old's wisdom

Toddler: Is it a good idea to use
spaghetti sauce as finger paint?

Magic 3 Ball:
Surprisingly, no.

Applesauce is a much better
medium to work with. Though
the hue is not as vibrant,
it smears on thicker
and allows you to
create a higher
level of art.

SPOTLIGHT:
THE FIVE-SECOND RULE

If you're living with a toddler, you know all about the "Five-Second Rule." If an item rests on the floor for less than five seconds, it's still OK to eat. But truth be told, it should be called the "Twenty-Second Rule." Here's why.

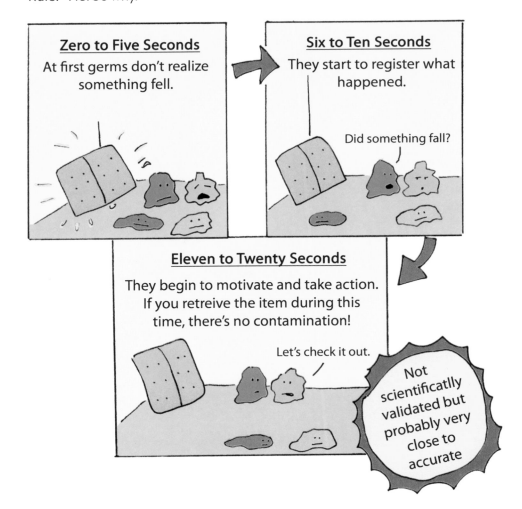

Zero to Five Seconds
At first germs don't realize something fell.

Six to Ten Seconds
They start to register what happened.

Did something fall?

Eleven to Twenty Seconds
They begin to motivate and take action. If you retreive the item during this time, there's no contamination!

Let's check it out.

Not scientificatlly validated but probably very close to accurate

THE COOKING NETWORK PRESENTS: TODDLER KITCHEN CREATIONS!

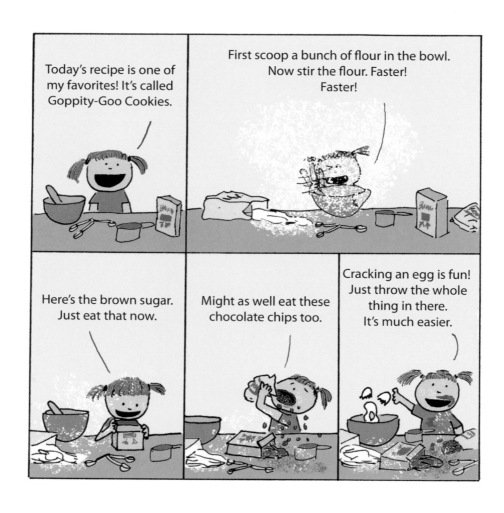

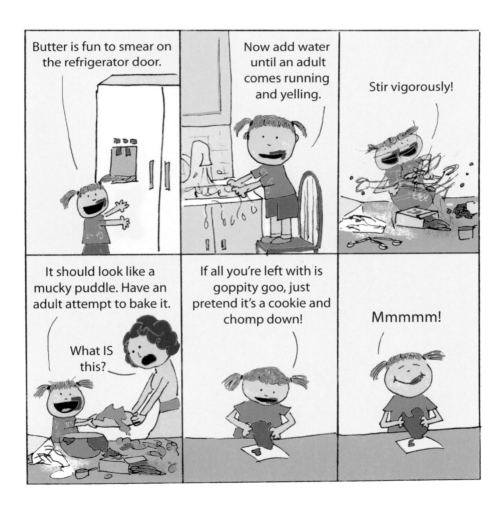

LOW MAINTENANCE!

Despite some high-maintenance tendencies, toddlers can also be extremely low maintenance. Consider the following:

1. They don't mind eating WALL*E toothpaste and ice for breakfast.

2. They sneeze on their food and just keep on eating.

3. Pasta with absolutely nothing on it? Yum!

4. They aren't embarrassed to wear bibs with sayings like "I pee in pools."

5. They like having food smeared all over clothes and face.

6. So what if it's a major social function, such as a wedding? The more food caked on Toddler's face, the cuter it is!

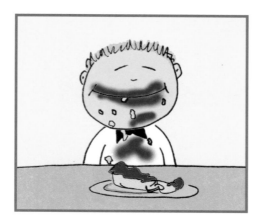

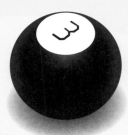

Ask the
Magic 3 Ball
Ask the Magic 3 Ball and
tap into a three-year-old's wisdom

Toddler: Is smearing peanut butter all over
my baby sister a good idea?

Magic 3 Ball:
No, take it
further.

Smearing peanut butter
and jelly and adding
bread is a better
approach.

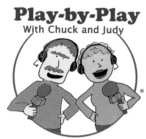

Play-by-Play
With Chuck and Judy

SNACK **TIME**

*Toddler wants a snack. How will this situation unfold?
Let's hear from our commentators, Chuck and Judy,
who are live on the scene with a play-by-play report.*

Chuck, Toddler wants a banana.

Judy, this is tense.

I know it.

Mom has the banana in hand. She's
watching for a sign that it's OK to peel.

There's the sign!

Peeling is under way. She needs to
keep this slow and controlled so she
can stop at exactly the right point.

Chuck, if she peels even a centimeter
too much, that banana is ruined.

That's right.

I think we all remember what happened
last week, when she pulled the
granola bar wrapper down too far.

And let's not forget the incident
with the string cheese wrapper.

What about the time Dad handed
Toddler a naked banana?

That was so outrageous. So emotional.

I think we're getting close . . . close.

NO!

She's stopping!

Whew! Right at the perfect point.
Chuck, this mom is finally getting it.

Finally!

Play-by-Play
With Chuck and Judy

Next: *Chuck and Judy are live from the scene of a playdate.*

NOTES FOR THE BABYSITTER

From the Desk of Toddler's Mommy

Dear Katie,

Thank you for babysitting for us today! We've jotted down a few notes about giving Bobby his snack. Best of luck!

Bobby eats his snack while watching his favorite train cartoon. Here are the steps you need to follow.

1. At 10:56, open the pantry door.

2. Extract a breakfast bar from the box; lay it on the counter, parallel to the phone. Do not open the wrapper yet!

3. Pick Bobby up and put him in his high chair.

4. Turn on the TV and exclaim "Choo-choo!" (Do not say "Woo-woo!" He'll be listening for that "ch" sound.)

5. Now unwrap the breakfast bar, discard the wrapper, and hand the bar to Bobby.

6. He will hold it up against his pursed lips as he waits for the show to begin.

From the Desk of Toddler's Mommy

7. Waiting . . . waiting . . .

8. When he hears the show's song, he will begin eating.

9. While he is eating his bar, cut up string cheese and strawberries. Put those on his tray.

10. When Bobby is done with his breakfast bar, he will start to slowly push the strawberries and cheese toward the edge of his tray. He will stare right at you as he does this.

11. Try to pay attention because if you don't dash over to him in time, he will push all the food off the edge and you'll have quite a mess to clean up.

12. Once he rejects the cheese and strawberries, Bobby will demand another breakfast bar. Firmly tell him no.

13. Be prepared for a very negative reaction.

See you later this afternoon. Don't call us; we'll call you!

A TODDLER'S IDEAL RESTAURANT

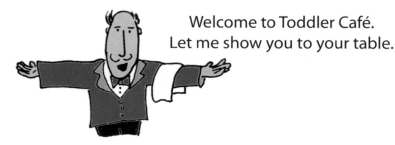

Welcome to Toddler Café.
Let me show you to your table.

What? No, no, no. There are no chairs here.
You simply wander around while you eat.
If you'd like to dine naked, that is
perfectly fine.

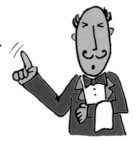

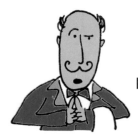

Napkins?
I'm afraid I dont know what you're talking about.

Our special tonight is fish. Goldfish crackers, to
be precise. Personally licked by the chef.

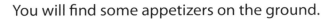

You will find some appetizers on the ground.

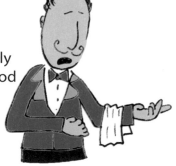

If you don't like your food, simply open your mouth and let the food fall out onto the table.

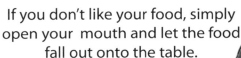

If you like the look of your neighbor's food, by all means steal it.

May I interest you in juice? Refills are immediate and endless.

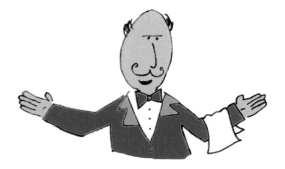

Oh yes: When you're done, let us know by vigorously wiping all the remaining food off your plate and onto the floor. Enjoy your meal!

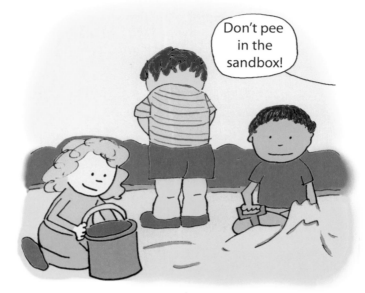

Chapter 3

The Social Lives of TODDLERS

Peeing in the sandbox. Though this violation might offend an adult during a social gathering, it's commonly accepted during a toddler's playdate. No feelings hurt. No friendships destroyed.

Let's take an inside look at how toddlers interact, play, share (yeah, right), and enjoy the company of others. Come, hop in the sandbox! (Just watch out for that wet spot.)

MYTH BUSTERS

There is a chasm between what adults and toddlers believe when it comes to play. Consider the following:

Parent myth: Educational toys provide a solid foundation of math, spelling, and geography skills.
Toddler truth: They also provide a physics tutorial—as in the force required to bash the gadget with a plastic hammer.

Parent myth: Blocks, dolls, and plastic trains are toys.
Toddler truth: "Toys" also come in the form of expensive lotion bottles, litter boxes, dust bunnies, and anything in Mom's purse.

Parent myth: It's best to put the board game pieces back in the board game box. We don't want to lose them.
Toddler truth: Put them back? Are you crazy?! They're going to be used as obstacles on the train track!

Parent myth: Expensive toys with bells and whistles will entertain Toddler for a long time.
Toddler truth: Please get this strange toy out of my face. All I really want to do is play with that stick on the ground. For an hour straight.

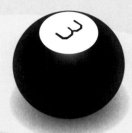

Ask the
Magic 3 Ball

Ask the Magic 3 Ball and
tap into a three-year-old's wisdom

Toddler: Would my daddy's wine bottles
make good bowling pins?

Magic 3 Ball:

Absolutely.

When you grow tired
of that, try them as
baseball bats.

IT WON'T BE PRETTY

Unless you have a college degree in mechanical engineering, don't expect to open a packaged toy without spilling some blood, testing the bounds of your patience, and exposing your child to some choice four-letter words.

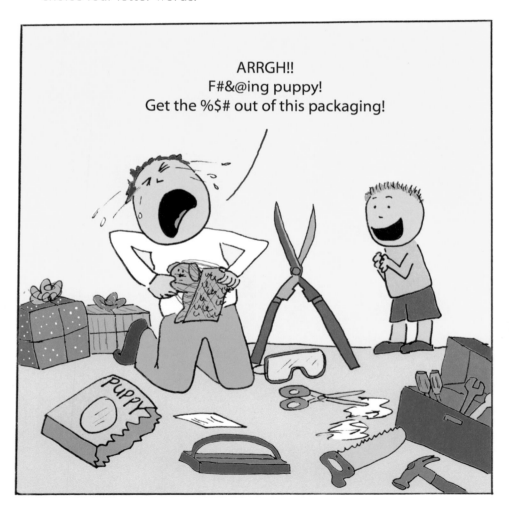

TODDLERS' FAVORITE GAMES

Your Turn!

How it works: You sit on the ground and your toddler rolls a ball toward you. It barely progresses past his foot. He yells, "Your turn!" forcing you to get up and retrieve the ball. You roll it to him. He accidentally rolls it off to a corner. And guess what: "Your turn!" again. Repeat until you can't take it any longer.

Better One or Two?

How it works: Your toddler asks you to undress a doll. You oblige. She studies the doll and is displeased. She asks you to redress it. You oblige. But this is not acceptable either. You are asked to undress the doll again. This dress-undress cycle continues until you have a mental breakdown.

One by One

How it works: Toddler is playing with a huge assortment of toy cars and other vehicles. When it's time to clean up, you dump a handful of vehicles in the toy bin. Toddler freaks out and dumps vehicles right back out. Then he begins putting them back the "right way." One . . . by . . . one. Slowly. Methodically. Examining each one as he goes. Don't worry; they'll all be put away. Four hours from now.

IN TO WIN

What would happen if toddlers wrote the instructions for competitive games? No matter the game, here's how the directions would read:

HOW TO PLAY

1 The only acceptable outcome of this game is for Toddler to win.

2 No ties, no multiple winners. Just Toddler winning. That is all.

3 Toddler reserves the right to change any rules, at any time.

4 If Toddler somehow loses, that means:

A the parents flagrantly cheated.

B and this game is totally unfair.

C and the past twenty minutes have been a complete waste of time.

D and this is too much to take. A tantrum must be performed.

TODDLER HANDBOOK
TIPS FOR TODDLERS, BY TODDLERS

TIPS FOR PLAYING HIDE AND SEEK

Tips If You Are the Counter

✏️ Attempt to count to twenty. If you can't get that far, just count to elleventeen.

✏️ If the anticipation is killing you, count to three and be done with it.

✏️ As you count, very subtly peek out through your fingers and look all around to see if you can determine where the hider is planning to go.

✏️ If, after ten seconds of seeking, you haven't found the hider, yell "Gimme hint!" or simply "Come out!"

Tips If You Are the Hider

✏️ Hide in the place where your parent just hid. Or keep hiding in the same place over and over.

✏️ When your parent yells, "Ready or not, here I come!" reveal yourself immediately.

✏️ If time is running out and you're getting flustered looking for a place to hide, just crouch in the middle of the room and cover your face with your hands. Remember: *If you can't see them, they can't see you.*

WHICH TODDLER TOY HAVE YOU MOST BONDED WITH?

You pick them up day in and day out. Even though it may drive you crazy, admit it—you have a soft spot in your heart for at least one of your toddler's toys. Which one exactly? Take this quiz and find out!

1. It's midmorning, and you have a neighbor unexpectedly drop by. What is the state of your front room?
   A. Piles everywhere. Organized piles, but piles nonetheless.
   B. Furniture has been rearranged by Toddler.
   C. A strange sticky film covers everything.

2. Ugh. Toddler wants mac and cheese again! What lunch would you give anything to share with your toddler?
   A. Triple-decker club sandwich
   B. An appetizer platter
   C. I don't eat lunch. I prefer to chew gum.

3. Which movie would you likely let Toddler watch first?
   A. **Sleepless in Seattle**: Seeing the Empire State Building scene makes you happy.
   B. **Freaky Friday**: You love how everything is all switched around.
   C. **Transformers**: You like the way they're always changing. It's a speedboat! Wait, it's a robot!

The Results

If you answered mostly:

As

You have a soft spot for . . . LEGOs.

LEGOs speak to you because you are the queen of piles. Odds are there's a stack of bills in your house so tall that you likely owe a magazine subscription payment from 1997. And did you have gravity-defying bangs in high school? We thought so.

Bs

You have a soft spot for . . . Mrs. Potato Head.

Like Mrs. Potato Head, you like to mix things up. So what if you wear a bandana as a bra or jogging shoes with a dress? Deal with it, people. At least you don't have an ear where your nose should be, right?

Cs

You have a soft spot for . . . Silly Putty.

You go with the flow, and can adapt to things easily, much like a ball of Silly Putty. Sometimes you get so into multitasking, you tend to bounce off the walls. If only you could crawl into a red eggshell at the end of the day and snap it shut . . .

ANATOMY OF A PLAY GROUP

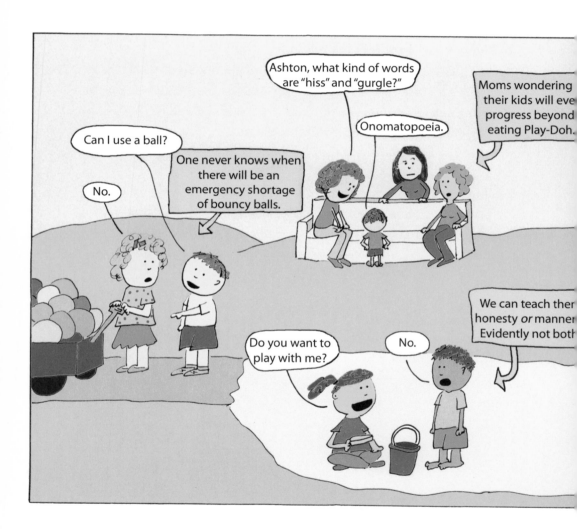

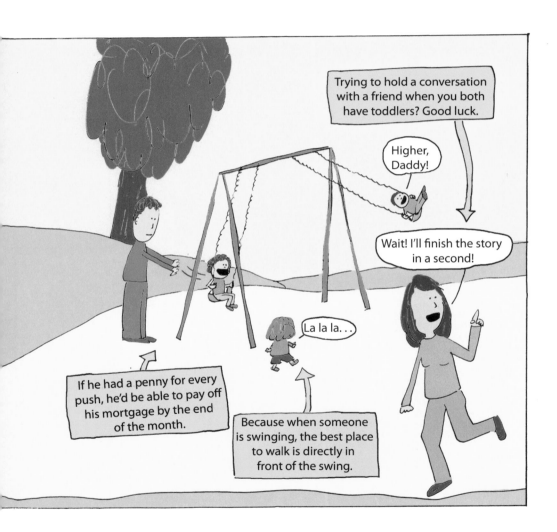

TODDLER YOGA MOVES

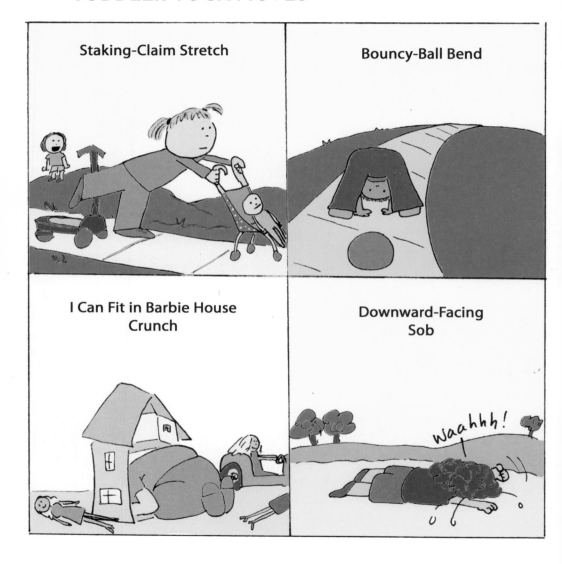

TODDLER HANDBOOK
TIPS FOR TODDLERS, BY TODDLERS

HOW TO PUT ON A FABULOUS SHOW

- Charge a lot for the tickets. Somewhere in the ballpark of a thousand hundred million dollars.

- When you sell the tickets, pretend to be someone else. This way your theater company appears to be larger than it actually is.

- Once everyone is seated, make a big production out of "getting ready for the show." The audience will wait it out while you elaborately prepare.

- Is it showtime and you have no ideas? Don't worry. Anything can be a show. Bobbing lightly to an entire Barney CD is a show. Fiddling with your fake vacuum cleaner is a show. Even standing there thinking about what to do for a show is a show.

- Keep your show going for at least two hours. Remember, these people paid a lot of money.

Play-by-Play
With Chuck and Judy

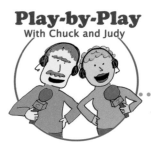

PARK TIME

A toddler playdate is forming at the park. Our commentators, Chuck and Judy, are live on the scene to give us a play-by-play report.

Judy, they've pulled up to the park.
Mom is opening the minivan door.

Whoa! Toddler is holding a huge pile of stuff on her lap. Look at that!

Mom is trying to get her to leave that stuff in the car.

That's not going to fly. Look, Toddler is climbing out of
the car, still holding on to all of her special things.

She's walking over to that tree. . . . Judy, I think she's just going
to stand next to the tree, holding her treasured toys.

Here comes Toddler's friend to say hi.

Oh! Toddler is shaking her head.
She's got a pretty hostile look on her face.

Here comes another friend to say hi.

That little head is still vehemently shaking no.

Mom is encouraging Toddler to play.

She can't be serious, Judy. Doesn't she know that
those kids will just steal Toddler's best toys?

That's right, Chuck. The point of bringing your toys to the park is
to stand there and hold them. Make sure no one else gets them.

Yes. Her plan is to hold tight and not move for
the entire ninety-minute playdate.

That's a great plan.

Remember the time she wanted to sit in the baby-
doll stroller during that other playdate? She just sat
and sat and sat. Over two hours of sitting.

It's too risky to even play with your things or
other kids might want to play, too.

All you can do is show up and guard your stuff.

Guard it with your life, Chuck.
Guard it with your life.

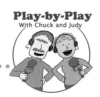

Play-by-Play
With Chuck and Judy

*Next: What happens when Toddler gets dressed? Chuck and
Judy report.*

CONFLICT RESOLUTION ACCORDING TO TODDLERS

We can coach toddlers on the "right way" to resolve problems, but chances are, they'll want to handle it their own way.

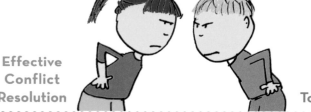

Effective Conflict Resolution	The Toddler Way
Maintaining a good relationship should be the first priority.	Priority = ME.
Listen first, talk second.	Best to skip straight to yelling and sobbing.
Agree on the facts.	That's easy: The fact is you wronged me. You wronged me bad.
Explore options together.	Your option is to surrender or get kicked in the shin.
Collaborate and compromise.	Blah, blah. These words don't even make sense.
Solve the issue.	A kick in the shin it is!

BEHIND THE WHEEL

You're doing some quick gardening in the front yard. A couple feet away, Toddler is quietly playing in your car. It's parked in the driveway, you have the keys, and the windows are rolled all the way down. Everything seems fine . . . until you attempt to drive somewhere later. Then you realize the many ways you paid for this peace and quiet.

- The radio blasts at maximum volume when you turn on the car.

- Your seat is moved so far up your chin is resting on the steering wheel.

- Windshield wipers start quickly swishing to and fro.

- Hazard lights are blinking.

- Battery is drained because light was left on.

- Crayon art decorates walls and ceiling.

- Every CD is missing but the cases are still there.

- Your day-old coffee is also missing.

- A coin is lodged in steering wheel shaft. Now, every time you turn left, your horn honks.

TA-DA!

From boring to fascinating, just like that!

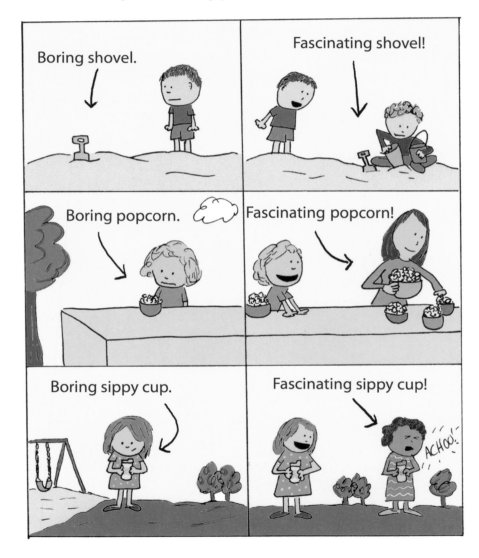

ROYAL FLUSH

During the toddler years, a lot of action takes place at the toilet. No, not potty training; throwing things in. From a toddler's viewpoint, the commode is one of the best toys around.

Give yourself:

1 point if Toddler has placed any of the following objects in the toilet

2 points if Toddler actually flushed them down

5 points if you succeeded in a search-and-rescue operation

• •

- DVD of *Finding Nemo*
- An actual goldfish
- A fish stick
- Pair of pajamas
- Kitchen utensil
- Box of crayons (bonus point if all crayons were recovered)
- An entire roll of toilet paper, including the tube
- Mobile phone
- Balloon
- Shampoo bottle
- Toddler's book about potty training
- Flashlight (still on)

• •

0–10 points: Not much potty play happening at your house!

11–20 points: Who needs Toys "R" Us? Just head to the toilet aisle at Home Depot for fun times!

More than 21 points: Impressive aqua rescue experience! You should enlist in the Navy Seals.

OK, THAT'S ENOUGH PRETEND

It's fun to watch your toddler play pretend. Until things start to sound a little too familiar.

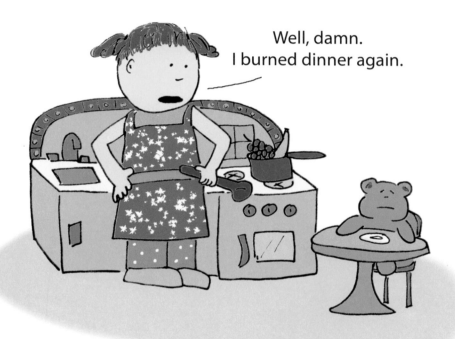

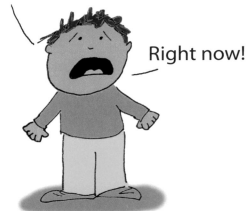

But Mommy!
I wannahhanaaaaah
gaaahmana flehmana!

Right now!

Chapter 4

Use Your WORDS

Few things are as amusing as a toddler talking. The way they piece sentences together, the way they mispronounce words, the way they make passionate declarations about everything around them: What's not to love?

Of course, you do run into the problem of them being a tad too honest at times. And since they can talk, they can also order you around. And negotiate. And question everything. And concoct crazy lies. And . . . well, maybe there are a *few* downsides.

Come, let's chat about talking.

TODDLER HANDBOOK
TIPS FOR TODDLERS, BY TODDLERS

HOW TO TALK

✏️ Stutter extensively. Start your sentence over at least five times.

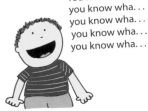

You know wha. . .
you know wha. . .
you know wha. . .
you know wha. . .
you know wha. . .

✏️ Talk about yourself in third person. It makes it easier for your parents to understand.

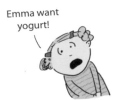

Emma want yogurt!

✐ The words "me" and "you" are completely interchangeable.

Pick you up?

✐ Say in a very whiny voice "Mommmmmy?" before starting any sentence.

Mommmmmmy!

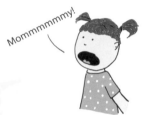

✐ Stick with your mom. She'll serve as your translator for the next few years.

Oodie foot!   He wants his shoes

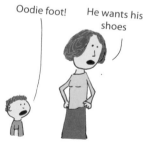

NEGOTIATION TIME

Toddlers are shrewd negotiators and never take "no" for an answer. Perhaps we should take a page from their playbook.

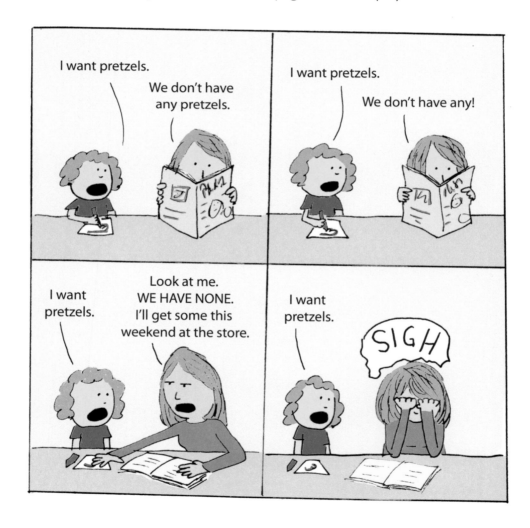

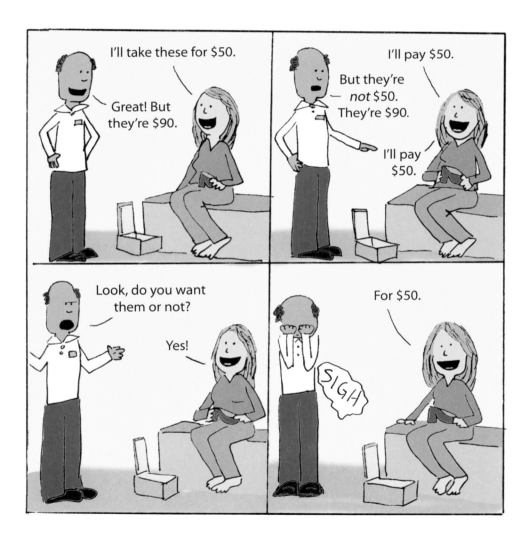

TODDLER HANDBOOK
TIPS FOR TODDLERS, BY TODDLERS

WORDS TO USE OFTEN

"Airplane! Look!"
Parents are notoriously oblivious to the miracles of aviation. Anytime you see a plane it is your duty to make sure they see it and appreciate it with a "Yay!" or light applause. This goes for helicopters as well.

"Best" / "Worst"
Things are either the "best ever" or "worst ever." There is no middle ground.

"Me do it!" / "Do it myself!"
If you're not saying this at least twenty times per hour, get with the program. You should be shouting it left and right, whether it's related to putting on your shoes or pulling the car into the garage.

"Mine"
Whatever you see is yours. Claim it.

"Mommy!"
Hungry, tired, uncomfortable, or bored? Yelling "Mommy!" is the remedy. If your mom doesn't immediately bend down and look directly at you, step up the intensity and the pace. "Mommy! Mommy! Mommy!" This rapid-fire repetition is especially good for a long car ride.

"No"

This powerful word is appropriate at any time, in any setting. In fact, you can keep repeating "No!" even as you are performing the task that was requested of you. This will let your parents know that your body may be obeying, but your mind is rebelling.

"One more time!"

Say this whenever something fun ends. Do not stop saying it until the fun thing starts again.

"Poop"

This word is completely hilarious and can be used over and over to demonstrate your incredible sense of humor. Also try "poopy head" or "poopy pants" or even "poopy pants mommy." For a funny observation, say "I see poop on your head!" or, simply, "Watch out for poop!" It will crack your friends up every time.

"The trash truck!"

Trash trucks are, in a word, incredible. Possibly more incredible than airplanes. Anytime you hear one, drop what you are doing, yell "The trash truck!" and take off for the front door. Watch the truck until it turns the corner and drives out of sight. Then insist on following it.

"Why?"

This should be the automatic response to any directions your parents give. You know you're on the right track if your mom yells, "Because I told you so!" or "Go ask your dad!" To which you should, of course, reply: "Why?"

TODDLER ON AISLE THREE

No one is quite sure why, but when toddlers enter a grocery store, they instantly become ten times more outlandish.

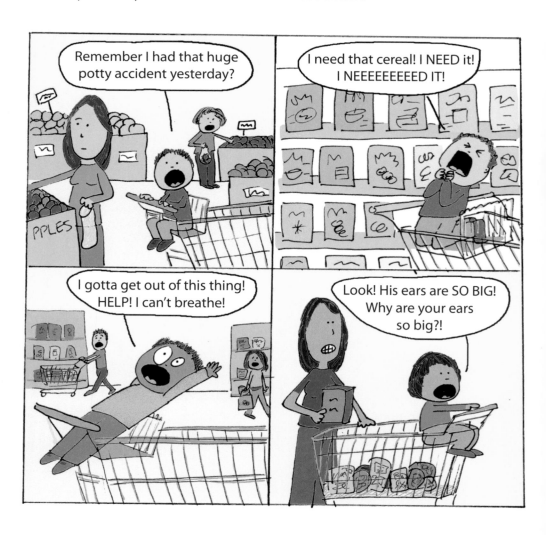

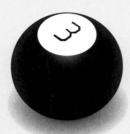

Ask the Magic 3 Ball

Ask the Magic 3 Ball and tap into a three-year-old's wisdom

Toddler: When my mom sticks the phone to my ear and my grandma asks me a question, can I just nod as a response?

Magic 3 Ball:
Definitely!

Grandma will hear you nodding through the phone. Also, if Mom hands you the phone and lets you hold it while Grandma is talking, be sure to wander off and hide the phone somewhere obscure. Don't hang up; just hide it.

THE TRUTH ABOUT LYING

Toddlers think that if they answer quickly with a lie, they will surely be believed, despite the content of what they're actually saying. Consider the following:

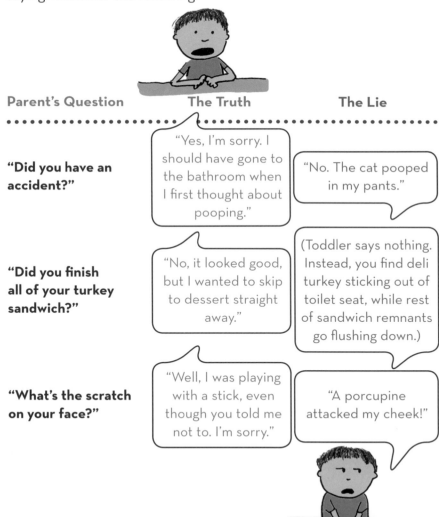

Parent's Question	The Truth	The Lie
"Did you have an accident?"	"Yes, I'm sorry. I should have gone to the bathroom when I first thought about pooping."	"No. The cat pooped in my pants."
"Did you finish all of your turkey sandwich?"	"No, it looked good, but I wanted to skip to dessert straight away."	(Toddler says nothing. Instead, you find deli turkey sticking out of toilet seat, while rest of sandwich remnants go flushing down.)
"What's the scratch on your face?"	"Well, I was playing with a stick, even though you told me not to. I'm sorry."	"A porcupine attacked my cheek!"

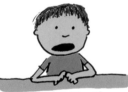

Parent's Question	The Truth	The Lie
"Why did you pull all the clothes out of your drawers?"	"It was an impulsive move, and I regret that it happened."	"That happened all by itself! I saw it happen all by itself!"
"Where's your cookie? Did you shove the whole thing in your mouth and swallow it already?!"	"Unfortunately, the answer is yes."	"No, Mama! I had to give it to a big team of skunks so they wouldn't spray me!"
"The TV is all messed up! Did you push a bunch of buttons on the remote?"	"I did. And believe me, I'm as upset as you are."	"A pirate ran in and did it. But don't worry—I punched him!"

TODDLER HANDBOOK

TIPS FOR TODDLERS, BY TODDLERS

HOW TO CARRY ON A GREAT CONVERSATION

Step One

To start a conversation, yell out the first thing that occurs to you. For example:

- ✎▷ "I have a cat!"

- ✎▷ "More juice!"

- ✎▷ "My daddy has no hair!"

Step Two

Someone may respond to you, but you don't need to listen to what they say. Just watch their mouth. When it stops moving (or if you anticipate that it will stop moving soon), yell out another random thought.

- ✎▷ "My bum has a rash on it!"

- ✎▷ "I can karate chop you!"

- ✎▷ "Give me a piggy back ride!"

Step Three

To close out a conversation, simply stand there and make a grimacing face, like you're pooping in your pants. (If you feel the need, you can actually poop.) This will more than likely end the conversation.

SPLIT PERSONALITY?

Is a close friend or relative coming for a social visit? Get ready to see two completely different sides of your toddler.

UH-OH

One thing to know about toddlers: It takes a lot to elicit an "uh-oh" out of them. If your toddler has been playing alone and suddenly you hear them shout those two words, prepare yourself. It won't be pretty.

Let's look at what it might take to get an "uh-oh" out of a toddler—and how that compares with parents.

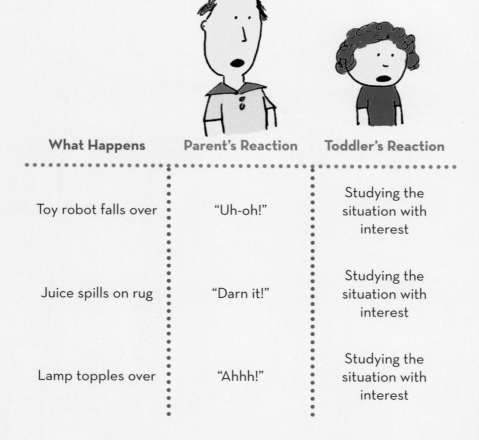

What Happens	Parent's Reaction	Toddler's Reaction
Toy robot falls over	"Uh-oh!"	Studying the situation with interest
Juice spills on rug	"Darn it!"	Studying the situation with interest
Lamp topples over	"Ahhh!"	Studying the situation with interest

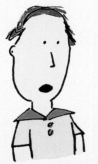
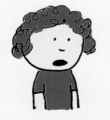

What Happens	Parent's Reaction	Toddler's Reaction
Yogurt spills on computer keyboard	"Oh no! No, no, no!"	Studying the situation with interest
Pancake inserted in DVD player	"It's ruined! It's ruined!"	Studying the situation with interest
Pack of coyotes tears through house	"What the—?!"	"Doggy!"
Huge boulder rolls into side of house, crushing an entire wall	"Call 911! Someone help!"	"Ball."
Backyard explodes and hot lava starts shooting out	"Run for your lives!"	"Uh-oh."

HIGH-TECH TODDLER

It's only a matter of time before toddlers jump on the social media bandwagon. What kind of profile pages would they have?

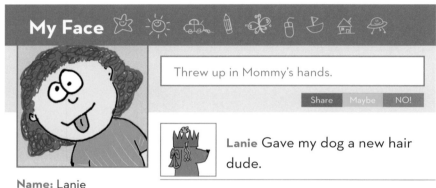

My Face

Threw up in Mommy's hands.

Share   Maybe   NO!

Lanie Gave my dog a new hair dude.

Lanie When can I stop taking naps already??

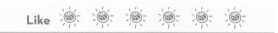

Like

Lanie No one except Mommy can read to me.

Dad Can't I read to you?

Lanie JUST MOMMY!

Lanie Mailman just delivered box full of Styrofoam "peanuts"! This is going to be an *awesome* day!

Name: Lanie

Friends: Six Friends

Groups: I Love String Cheese, Twelve Hours of TV Isn't Bad for You

Interested in: Twirling

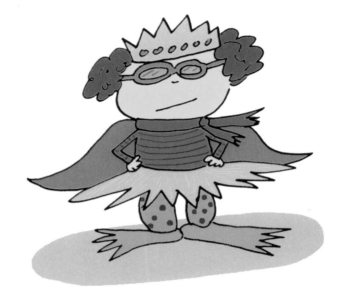

Chapter 5

GROOMING

Is it easy to keep toddlers looking sharp? No. Not at all.

They resist the hairbrush. They are scared of the bath. And they develop zealous, unyielding preferences for clothing color, fit, style, fabric, and licensed characters.

Of course, for many toddlers, *nudity* is the only true option to be entertained.

Why all the drama? Let's head into the world of grooming and find out.

Toddler Handbook
Tips for Toddlers, by Toddlers

FASHION MUSTS

✏️ The proper way to wear underwear is *backward*.

✏️ If you wear diapers, they must be put on while you are *standing up*.

✏️ Think of a signature trademark, such as a flower pattern, twirly skirts, or clothing featuring fire engines. Once you pick one, that's it. Your clothing *must* conform or you will not wear it.

✏️ There is no such thing as "clashing hues."

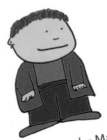

Red + red + red = Match

✏️ There is no such thing as clothes that are "inside out."

✏️ There is no such thing as "dirty clothes" or "clothes that are in the laundry."

✏️▷ There is no such thing as "clashing patterns."

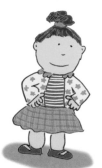

Flowers complement stripes which complement plaid

✏️▷ Pajamas are clothes. They count as "being dressed."

✏️▷ Your parents will talk about "right shoe" and "left shoe." Ignore them. Any shoe can be worn on any foot.

✏️▷ Any size shoe is also acceptable.

✏️▷ Refuse the jacket. You will not get cold.

TODDLER'S OUTFIT: PREDICT RIDICULOUSNESS

Begin with 10 points. (The baseline absurdity level of any toddler outfit.)

__ Is Dad in charge of dressing Toddler? Add 100 points.

__ Are you under a time crunch? Add 200 points.

__ Is Toddler currently wearing favorite pajamas? Add 50 points.

__ Is there a pair of inappropriate shoes (for example, special occasion shoes, snow boots) within Toddler's sight? Add 50 points.

__ Is there a tutu and/or superhero cape nearby? Add 75 points.

__ Is Toddler in a "pretending to be a doggy" phase and currently wearing yarn tail fastened by piece of scotch tape? Add 60 points.

__ Is Toddler unusually strong and prone to wild kicking? Add 40 points.

__ Is Toddler's favorite clothing item so dirty that it could be mistaken as a mound of topsoil? Add 60 points.

• •

Results: **How Ridiculous Will the Outfit Be?**

10–250 points = Passable

Sweats with patent leather shoes and no shirt? Go with it, and count your blessings.

251–450 points = Hmm

Even Lady Gaga would be hard pressed to dream up an outfit this bizarre.

451 or more = Unbelievable

"Unbelievable" is the only word to describe the look Toddler is sporting. Nudity may be a better option if the weather agrees.

OUTFIT SELECTION

Is Toddler selecting an outfit? Use this chart to see what you're in for.

Not Appropriate for Weather

Not Appropriate for Event

Not Matching At All

Outfit Toddler will want to wear to family reunion beach BBQ event

Toddler's Preferred Daily Outfit

Outfit Toddler will demand to wear on first day of preschool

Outfit Toddler will insist on wearing in the formal family portrait

AND THE WINNER IS . . .

Your toddler's preferred daily outfit will not involve any of the adorable new shirts that you bought. Nor will it involve the new pants or cute little shoes. No, all these clothing items will remain nicely organized in the closet, collecting dust.

Meanwhile, an old ratty clothing item will be the *sole acceptable garment*. And it will emerge the victor day after day after day after day. . . .

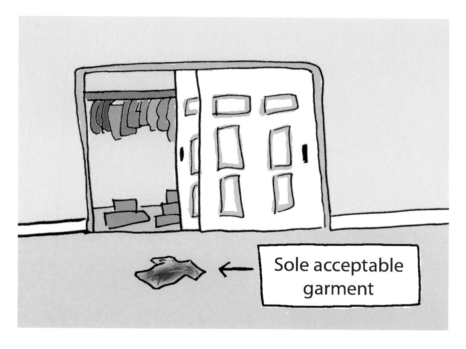

Sole acceptable garment

GETTING TODDLER DRESSED

Let's review the complicated dance known as "Getting Toddler Dressed."

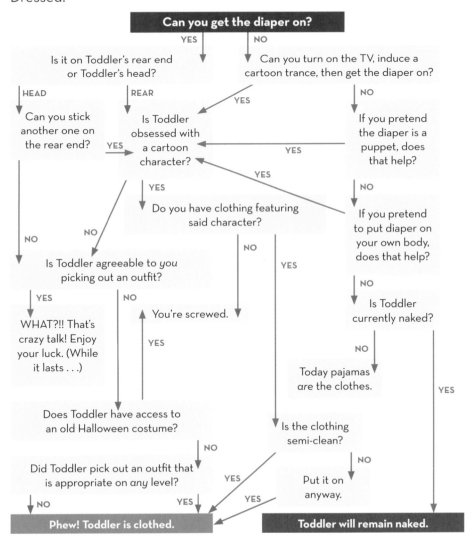

Can you get the diaper on?

YES → Is it on Toddler's rear end or Toddler's head?

- HEAD → Can you stick another one on the rear end?
  - NO →
  - YES → WHAT?!! That's crazy talk! Enjoy your luck. (While it lasts . . .)
- REAR → Is Toddler obsessed with a cartoon character?

NO → Can you turn on the TV, induce a cartoon trance, then get the diaper on?

- YES → Is Toddler obsessed with a cartoon character?
- NO → If you pretend the diaper is a puppet, does that help?
  - YES → Is Toddler obsessed with a cartoon character?
  - NO → If you pretend to put diaper on your own body, does that help?
    - YES → Is Toddler obsessed with a cartoon character?
    - NO → Is Toddler currently naked?
      - NO → Today pajamas are the clothes.
      - YES → **Toddler will remain naked.**

Is Toddler obsessed with a cartoon character?
- YES → Do you have clothing featuring said character?
  - YES → Is the clothing semi-clean?
    - YES → **Phew! Toddler is clothed.**
    - NO → Put it on anyway. → **Toddler will remain naked.**
  - NO → You're screwed.
- NO → Is Toddler agreeable to *you* picking out an outfit?
  - YES → Does Toddler have access to an old Halloween costume?
  - NO → Does Toddler have access to an old Halloween costume?

You're screwed. → YES → Does Toddler have access to an old Halloween costume?

Does Toddler have access to an old Halloween costume?
- NO → Did Toddler pick out an outfit that is appropriate on *any* level?
  - NO → **Phew! Toddler is clothed.**
  - YES → **Phew! Toddler is clothed.**
- YES → **Phew! Toddler is clothed.**

Today pajamas are the clothes. → Is the clothing semi-clean?

Play-by-Play
With Chuck and Judy

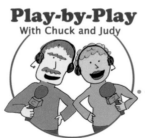

THE PERFECT ACCESSORY

Toddler has finally picked an outfit, and now has her eye on an accessory. Let's get the play-by-play report from our commentators, Chuck and Judy, who are live on the scene.

Chuck, Toddler is dressed, but I sense that something's missing.

Judy, I agree.

It looks like she's reaching up to get something on that shelf.

A box of Band-Aids. Brilliant.

Absolutely. This is the right move.

Judy, she went for three Band-Aids yesterday.
What do you think we'll see today?

Well, she needs one right above her upper lip for sure.

Yes. She does have a small "owie" on her nose, but as we saw yesterday she prefers to put the Band-Aid above her lip instead.

Well, that's close enough to the nose.

It sure is.

I believe we'll see some bandaging of the arms and legs today.

No "owies" there; instead, the Band-Aid is purely an accessory.

Chuck, she knows all the other toddlers will want this look.

Goodness, yes. Fortunately Mom bought those princess Band-Aids, and not the totally unacceptable plain Band-Aids, like before.

Yes, and this time the box was more accessible. Remember when it used to be stored way up in that cabinet?

Ironically, Toddler kept injuring herself just trying to get to the Band-Aids.

Here she goes . . . two, no, three bandages on the arms!

Now she's dumping them all out. Holding them up to the light so she can pick just the right princess.

Judy, I think she's really going for it. I think she is going to use them all.

Chuck, it's impossible to have too many.

Play-by-Play
With Chuck and Judy

Next: Toddler on an airplane. Chuck and Judy report.

LATE = NOT GREAT

Running late? Brace yourself. Toddler is sure to appear in the hallway wearing an outrageous outfit. The later you're running, the more absurd it will be.

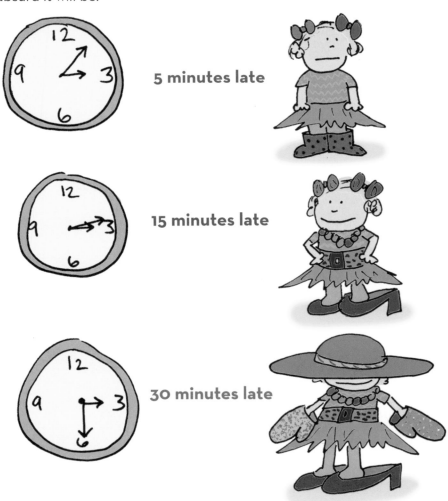

5 minutes late

15 minutes late

30 minutes late

AND . . . THERE IT IS

Did you know it takes approximately fourteen seconds for a new white shirt to get stained? Even if Toddler just stands there.

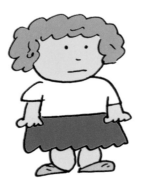

No stain

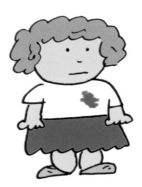

Stain

Time elapsed:
14 seconds

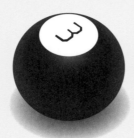

Ask the Magic 3 Ball

Ask the Magic 3 Ball and
tap into a three-year-old's wisdom

Toddler: Should I put on Mom's underwear
over my pants for Thanksgiving dinner and surprise
the entire family with my new look?

Magic 3 Ball:
Absolutely.

Find the largest, oldest pair of
underpants possible. If you
can somehow manage
to arrange her bra
on your head as
earmuffs, even
better.

HAIRCUT OR HORROR FILM?

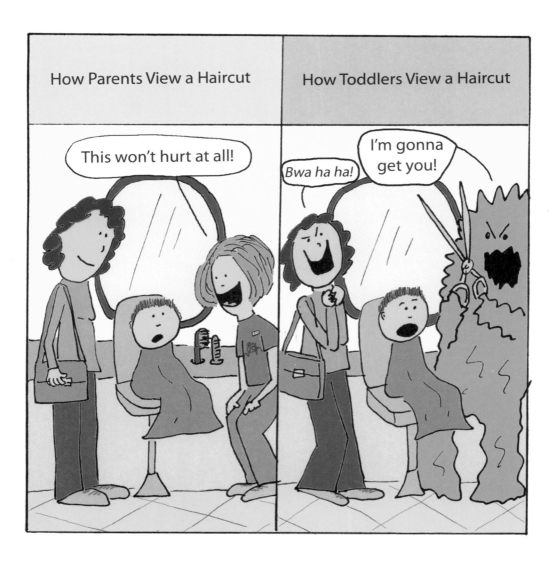

TODDLER HANDBOOK
TIPS FOR TODDLERS, BY TODDLERS

BATH RULES

- Remain standing at all times.

- Insist on bubbles. Lots and lots of bubbles.

- Make a choice: Either do not let water touch your face, or jump so hard in the tub that water splashes everywhere.

- Remove any product that is not a plastic toy from the tub by hurling it across the room, preferably in the direction of the toilet.

- If you get your hands on the soap or expensive shampoo bottle, squeeze the contents into the bathwater.

- Stay in until your toes have shriveled into tiny raisins and are no longer recognizable as toes.

- Without warning, get out and run around dripping wet.

- The only permissible towel is the one with the froggy hood.

TOOTHBRUSHING RULES

- Insist on holding the toothbrush. If your parents produce another toothbrush, insist on holding that one, too.

- Suck the toothpaste off immediately and swallow it.

- Demand more toothpaste.

- Repeat step 2.

- Chew on the toothbrush.

- Beware: Your parents will try to use the "it's my turn to brush your teeth" ploy. Do not fall for this. It is never the parent's turn.

- If your parent grabs the toothbrush and tries to take over, seal your lips and dodge the toothbrush by turning your head left and right, left and right. Continue until your parent surrenders.

- Floss is best used as fishing wire—to catch pretend fish in the toilet.

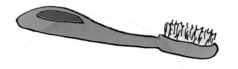

TODDLER HAIRSTYLES
AND WHAT THEY MEAN

Barrette basket is now empty.

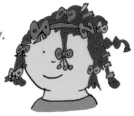

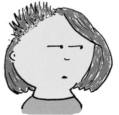

Scissors were left out.

Parents firmly believe there
is always enough hair for a
pony tail.

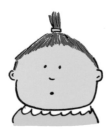

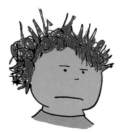

Hair-brush-phobia

Unauthorized use of
parents' hair gel.

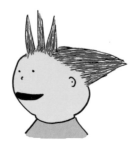

Chapter 6

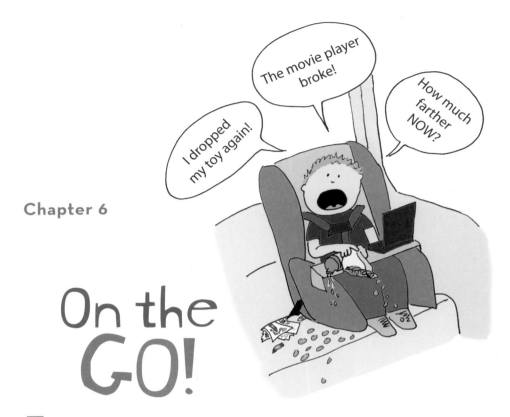

On the GO!

For adults, transportation is simple. It's about getting from *here* to *there*.

For toddlers, it's yet another opportunity to see how much power they wield—whether they're demanding outrageously crumbly snacks in the car, testing your patience with a road trip playlist of only three songs, or forcing you to change a dirty diaper in the middle of a desert.

Strap yourself in! We're about to explore toddlers and transportation.

TODDLER HANDBOOK

TIPS FOR TODDLERS, BY TODDLERS

GETTING READY TO LEAVE YOUR HOUSE

- If it's time to depart, do not rush. Take it slow; think about anything you might be forgetting, such as that miniature coloring book you got in that goodie bag four months ago. You're going to need that thing before anyone even *thinks* of leaving this house.

- Don't forget your entourage: your blankie, stuffed giraffe, pacifier, snack, magnetic drawing toy, pillow, other snack, favorite socks. Someone should start gathering all that stuff while you wait.

- Remember: It should not take any time to get to your destination. Zero minutes. So as soon as you are strapped into your car seat, ask your parents, "Are we there yet?"

LA RÉSISTANCE

Toddlers follow their own agendas when it comes to getting in the car seat. Which of the following have you experienced?

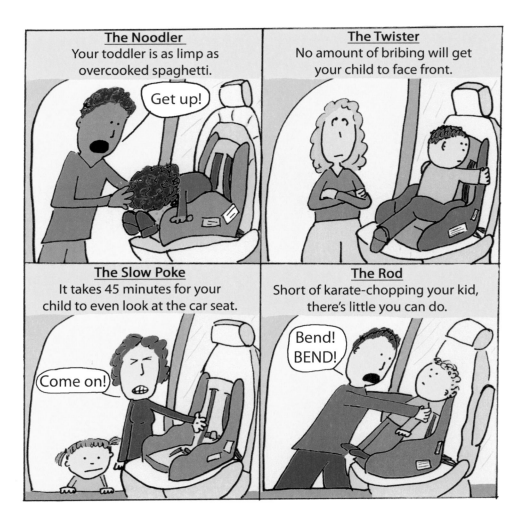

ME DO IT!

If you hear the words "Me do it!" accept that you will be very, very late to wherever you are going.

Here's how the extra time will likely break down:

- **Thirty minutes:** Toddler trying to heave his little body into your car.

- **Ten minutes:** Toddler getting situated in the car seat.

- **Twenty minutes:** Toddler trying to find all the straps, not realizing he's sitting on two of them.

- **Thirty minutes:** Toddler trying to fit one end of the chest buckle into the other end.

- **Five hours:** Toddler fumbling to buckle the lower buckle.

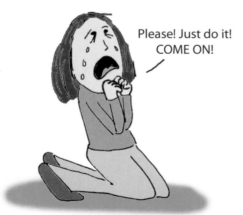

Please! Just do it!
COME ON!

Important: If you attempt to help in *any way,* you will contaminate the entire experience, and Toddler will need to start over from the "heaving self into car" step.

If you begin sobbing, don't worry. You are 100 percent normal.

WHICH OF THE FOLLOWING CAN YOU FIND IN YOUR CAR?

Make no mistake: The journey through toddlerhood takes a major toll on your car. Take a glance around and put a check by any of the following you spot:

☐ Cracker crumbs

☐ Random body part of toy

☐ Package of wipes open and dried out

☐ Backseat window adorned with boogers, fingerprints, and stickers

☐ At least eight CDs that contain cartoon voices

☐ Four CDs that you like but can no longer play because they are covered with unidentified sticky goo

☐ A mark on the exterior where Toddler kissed the dirty window

☐ Three different single shoes

☐ Old sippy cup with petrified beverage

☐ The reusable grocery bags that you never remember to bring into the store

☐ Halloween costume

☐ Handful of coffee stirrers Toddler snagged from Starbucks

☐ Detailed grocery list you needed last week

☐ Emergency stash of size 1 diapers, long forgotten

HOME

You put on Toddler's favorite CD. All is well.

Toddler requests "It's Great to Be an Engine" for twenty-second time. Help!

Yuck! Toddler poops in diaper, and there's no exit for twenty-nine miles. Plus, it's too cold to roll down the window.

Whew! Toddler remained calm and quiet during an important phone call. There's only one more phone call you need to make.

Oh no! Now she won't stop singing "I'm the Map" at the top of her lungs during your second call.

Ahhhh . . . so cute. Your little one says, "Mommy, hold my hand?" in the sweetest voice ever.

Uh-oh. You just ran out of snacks.

Yippie! You find snacks for starving Toddler stashed in your console. Do Fruit Roll-Ups expire?

A DRIVING WE WILL GO

What's it like to take a car trip with your toddler? Let's take a look.

You manage to stretch in an unfathomable yoga position to reach an all-important toy in the backseat, while keeping eyes on the road.

Ugh! Toddler just fell asleep two minutes from your destination. Wake up! Wake up!

You arrive at the baby shower you're cohosting. Should you drive back home so Toddler can get a full nap, or risk irritating your friend?

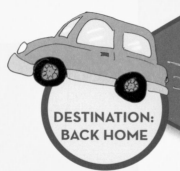

DESTINATION: BACK HOME

OUR WORLD, THEIR WORLD

When we were little, the World of Toddlers was a bit different. Let's look back . . .

Our Toddler World	Their Toddler World
Sitting on front seat arm rest during car ride or rolling around in the "back back"	Tightly strapped down in five-point harnessed, ergonomic car seat. Click, click, click, click, click!
Munching on granola bars, holding drink between legs	Enjoying prepackaged, organic, on-the-go yogurt packs and vitamin water boxes. Oh look, two cup holders! Excellent.
Quarreling with family members over which cassette to play	Each family member should be listening to his or her *own* iPod. And what's a cassette anyway?
Watching the full-service gas station attendant clean the windows	Watching a DVD from the ceiling of the minivan
Fighting with sibling. "He's on my side! She's touching me!"	OK, fine. This one is timeless.

1979

Today

Toddler Handbook
Tips for Toddlers, by Toddlers

STROLLER TIPS

◉▷ Understand this: You do not need a stroller. Your mom thinks you still need one, but she is dead wrong.

◉▷ If you are forced into a stroller, try to stand.

◉▷ As you are being pushed along, drop your toy at least three times.

◉▷ Situate your blankie so it is lightly dragging on the ground and in danger of being caught up in the wheel.

◉▷ At some point, insist on pushing your own stroller. The response will be "No." Keep insisting until you wear your parents down.

◉▷ When you are pushing your own stroller, you won't be able to see above the top of it. Don't worry. Push with confidence and let your instincts guide you.

◉▷ Accept no help with pushing the stroller.

◉▷ Once you've pushed the stroller, never go back to riding in the stroller. The only acceptable use of the stroller now is for you to push it.

PACKED UP!

Going on a trip? Be sure you follow the "Toddler World" guidelines when it comes to packing.

Ninety-six percent: Four times the diapers and wipes you'll actually need, six stuffed animals, three blankets, mismatched pair of light-up slippers, galaxy night-light machine, a tacklebox full of barrettes, SpongeBob toothpaste, Dora toothpaste, Spiderman toothpaste, favorite pillow, thirty books that Toddler picked out, enormous bag of LEGOs.

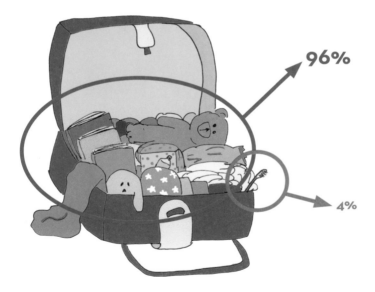

96%

4%

Four percent: Your extra pair of sweats, a toothbrush, and—if you're lucky—an extra hair band

SO SORRY

There are two words you'll undoubtedly say anytime you travel with toddler: "I'm sorry." Why not be proactive and get the apologies out of the way ahead of time? Simply hand these out:

Dear Fellow Travelers in Airport Security Line,
A warning: you may tear up when you watch my toddler wail in frantic sobs as she is forced to place her precious blanket through the x-ray machine. She may also turn and hit you in fury as we place the DVD Player on the belt. And plan on at least 23 minutes of wait time as she freaks out about walking through the metal detector. Oh, if you're able to help fold/unfold strollers and take out all of the liquids/creams from the diaper bag, that would be super. Might bring that wait time down to about 18 minutes.

Dear Surrounding Airline Passengers,
I apologize in advance if my toddler pokes at your ear, rips out the last pages of your mystery novel, stares directly at you for forty minutes straight, or asks you every thirty-eight seconds why you have no hair. Please, feel free to take my pretzels in exchange for any emotional damages caused.

Dear Person on the Street,

First, it's been a pleasure visiting your lovely city. Second, I am sorry that my toddler keeps walking very slowly right in front of you. You can try to get around her, but it's no use; she'll just adjust course and remain directly in front of you. She will probably stop abruptly several times as well. I would pull her out of the way, but honestly she is a ticking time bomb right now. (It's been a no-nap day!) Anyway, thank you for understanding. I'll just be right next to you, walking very slowly as well, if you have any questions.

Dear Hotel Guests,

Did you by chance hear some ear-piercing shrieking last night as I chased my toddler down the hallway at 4:30 a.m.? Sorry. We were only trying to get to the vending machine, where he pushed buttons until daybreak. Oh yes, and I hope you took extra vitamin C today, because my sniffly toddler also touched every piece of fruit and baked good in the free breakfast buffet. I think that covers things for now.

Play-by-Play
With Chuck and Judy

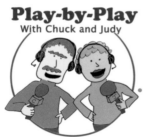

FLIGHT TIME

Toddler is on a plane. Let's find out how it's going. Our commentators, Chuck and Judy, are live on the scene with a play-by-play report.

Judy, Toddler seems a little bored sitting there in that enormous airplane seat.

Chuck, you got that right.

Mom is trying to get him to look at one of the toys she brought.

Well, Toddler already played with all those toys. He spent a good thirty seconds with each one. What else does she expect?

If she wanted him to be entertained for more than ten minutes she should have brought way more toys.

Exactly.

Looks like he's slowly sliding off the seat.

And . . . there he goes.

Ah! Mom is trying to pull him back up.

He's like a sack of potatoes.

Not budging at all.

Looks like Mom is telling him that the pilot has
turned on the fasten seatbelt sign.

Sign, shmine. She can't honestly expect Toddler to respond
to some "sign" that a "pilot" decided to "turn on."

You got that right, Chuck. No one is the boss
of this little guy. Not even the pilot.

Not even God.

Nope.

Oh, look. Toddler just stood up. He's starting to bang his
head against the back of that seat in front of him.

Whoa! That man just turned around and asked
Toddler to stop. What's that guy's problem?

The chair is right there. Of course Toddler
is going to bang his head on it.

It's got a big tray on it, too. You're telling me that Toddler isn't
allow to open and close that tray repeatedly for forty-five minutes
straight? If that's the case, why even put the tray there at all?!

Judy, what has air travel come to?

I don't know, Chuck. I don't know.

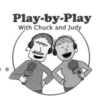

Play-by-Play
With Chuck and Judy

*Next: Unwrapping gifts can be an emotional rollercoaster.
Chuck and Judy file a report from the scene.*

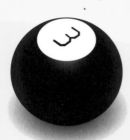

Ask the Magic 3 Ball

Ask the Magic 3 Ball and
tap into a three-year-old's wisdom

Toddler: When on vacation, is it acceptable to force
my parents to change my diaper on a sandy beach?

Magic 3 Ball:
Absolutely.

Make sure to roll off the diaper pad and get
sand all over your cracks and crevices.
Ideally there will be remnants of
poop on your bum as well, and
the sand will stick to that.
You don't get a diaper
change on the beach
very often, so
make the most
of it!

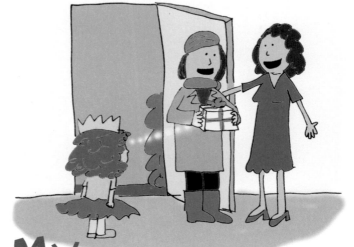

Chapter 7

Where's My PRESENT?

a.k.a. Birthdays and Holidays

Holidays. Birthdays. Special occasions. Those wonderful times when families get together to give, share, and enjoy one another. Who could ask for more?

Toddlers, that's who. And the specific question they're asking is this: "What's in it for me?"

From birthday party meltdowns to Halloween sugar highs and scary Santa encounters, toddlers make it through the holidays by remaining focused on the important things: gifts, candy, and more gifts.

Let's unwrap the toddler's worldview of special occasions!

BIRTHDAYS

If Toddlers Made Their Own Birthday Invitations

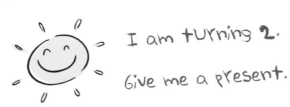

I am turning 2.

Give me a present.

I will tell you what I like.
I like trucks, drums,
Fig Newtons, and mud.

Do not come inside my house
because everything here
is for me. I do not want
to share my cake, and I
do not want to share my
party. Again, do not come
inside my house.

Bring the present and
then run away.

Party Planning

How do you plan a toddler's perfect birthday party? Chances are, your list of action items will be long and involved. Maybe you should consider thinking like a toddler instead.

Your view of what makes a great party:

Your toddler's view:

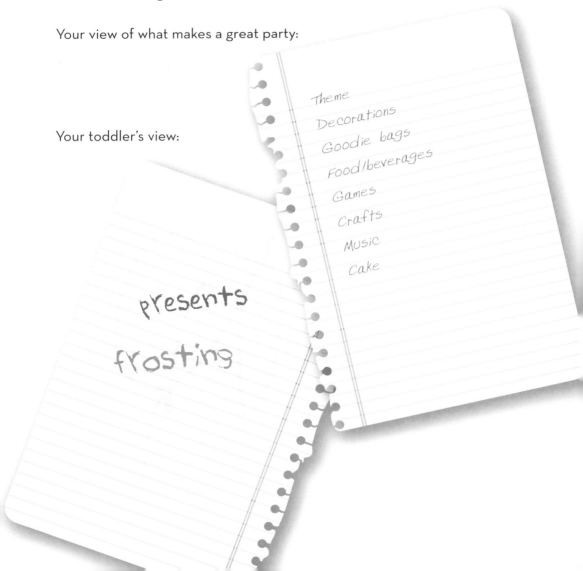

Theme
Decorations
Goodie bags
Food/beverages
Games
Crafts
Music
Cake

presents

frosting

Bigger, Better, Faster

Face painting? Please. That's so "First Birthday." Now that you have a toddler, it's time to step up the action. Just choose one from each of the columns to come up with an amazing birthday party plan.

Choose one from Column A	Choose one from Column B	Choose one from Column C
Zoo animals	waterskiing	on a roller coaster
Actual princess	break-dancing	with fireworks show
John Deere tractors	hula hooping	with a real dinosaur fossil
Nickelodeon stars	bungee jumping	with a rainbow in the sky
World-record hot dog eater	snake charming	in a horse-drawn carriage
Tightrope walker	driving ATV	on fake snow
Ice sculptor	skydiving	into pool full of doughnuts
Tarantulas	demolishing a building	with every Disney princess
Olympic medalist	telling your future	under a waterfall made of grape juice
Candy inventor	wrestling an alligator	covered in icing

Toddler Handbook
TIPS FOR TODDLERS, BY TODDLERS

PROPER SOCIAL SKILLS AT A BIRTHDAY PARTY

- During the "Happy Birthday" song you should sit directly in front of the cake and blow the candles out—no matter whose birthday is being celebrated.

- Attempt to stick your finger in the cake and/or remove one of the decorative items on the cake. You may be stopped, but it is at least polite to try.

- As soon as the hostess starts cutting the cake, begin yelling "I want cake! I want cake!" All the other kids will join you. Don't stop yelling until you have cake in hand.

- If you learn that you are going to receive a goodie bag at the end of the party, shout, "I want to leave right now!"

- If the goodie bags are different in any way, loudly complain that you want the other one.

- Upon receiving the goodie bag, dig through it and make critical observations. It's the only way the hostess will learn how to improve goodie bags in the future.

Opening Gifts at the Party: Always a Mistake

It's not a question of *if* the gift opening will go awry; it's a question of how disastrous it will be—and whether it will force you to immediately adjourn the party. See how your experience measures up.

Situation could be saved

Kids scoot *way* in to see what toddler is opening. One guest starts crying after getting squished.

Toddler is tearing through gifts with lightning speed, not slowing down to look at handmade cards or say thank you.

Toddler repeatedly yells, "I don't like this!" and "I already have this!"

Other kids start to "help" your toddler open gifts.

Other kids start to play with opened toys.

A new toy breaks.

Toddler is losing grip on emotions; full-blown tantrum is imminent.

Physical violence breaks out in the huddle; fists flying, tears flowing.

Party adjourned!

SEEMED LIKE A GOOD IDEA . . .

A piñata seems like a fun and exciting addition to a birthday party. But when you're dealing with toddlers, it never quite works out the way you planned. Here's how it usually goes down.

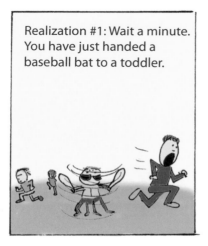

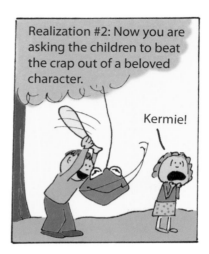

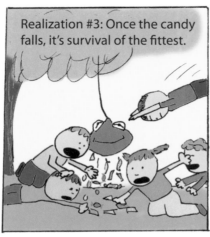

HOLIDAYS

The Lineup

How toddlers view holiday characters.

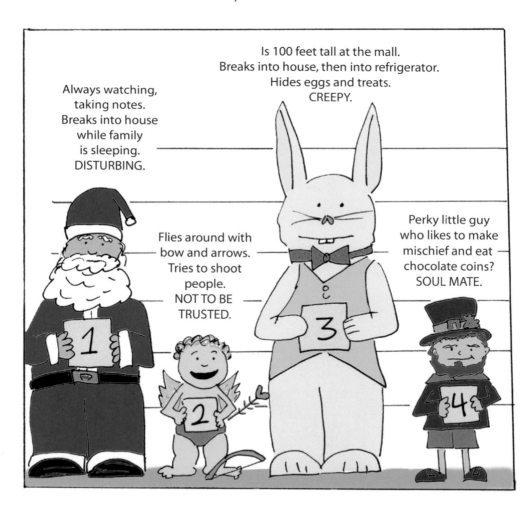

Always watching,
taking notes.
Breaks into house
while family
is sleeping.
DISTURBING.

Is 100 feet tall at the mall.
Breaks into house, then into refrigerator.
Hides eggs and treats.
CREEPY.

Flies around with
bow and arrows.
Tries to shoot
people.
NOT TO BE
TRUSTED.

Perky little guy
who likes to make
mischief and eat
chocolate coins?
SOUL MATE.

What the . . . ?

Match the expression to the toddler action.

She begs to be a vampire chinchilla for Halloween . . . and she insists *you* make the costume.

He announces he just found and ate the last Easter egg . . . and Easter was three weeks ago.

She pleads for a faster computer for Christmas, preferably with a 5G infranetwork.

He lets the family know at Thanksgiving dinner he's thankful he didn't drink *all* of the pee in the bathtub.

She wants a Rapunzel birthday cake and insists it has real hair.

Thanksgiving Dinner, the Toddler Version

Mmm! So much wonderful food is being prepared for Thanksgiving dinner! Alas, Toddler has ideas of his own.

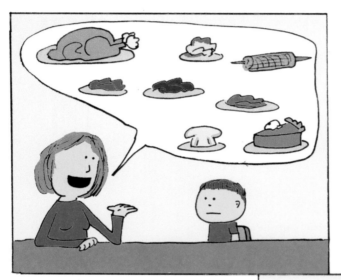

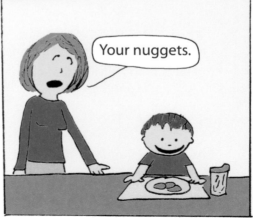

Toddler Handbook
TIPS FOR TODDLERS, BY TODDLERS

TOP FIVE EASTER RULES

- If you are dying eggs, the color should come out precisely as you imagined.

- The fake grass in your Easter basket does not belong in the basket. It belongs all over the house. So get to work.

- During the egg hunt, you should not be expected to exert undue effort. If you happen upon any egg that is even slightly out of your reach, order your parents to retrieve it. That's what they're there for.

- The proper way to eat a chocolate bunny is to sit in the sun and take your time. Let the bunny slowly melt all over your hands, face, and Easter outfit.

- You must, at some point, try to put a plastic egg back together. Use the two "bottom" halves of the eggs. (Do not use a bottom and top!) Keep working to fit the halves together, no matter how long it takes or how frustrating it becomes.

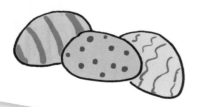

Time Warp

Every toddler knows that costumes aren't just for Halloween; they're appropriate on any day, no matter what the weather or occasion. In many cases, a costume will morph over the course of the year, as Toddler's tastes and interests change. For example:

Boy

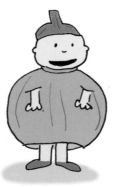

Pumpkin

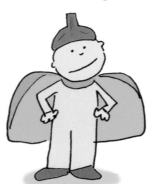

Superhero

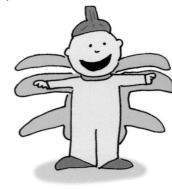

Spider

Girl

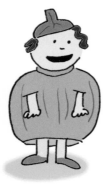

Pumpkin

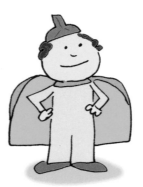

Superhero

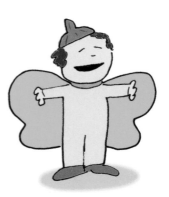

Butterfly

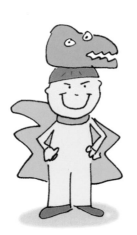

Dinosaur

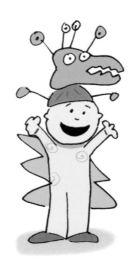

Alien Dinosaur

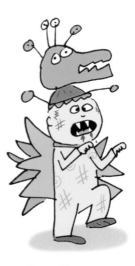

Alien Dinosaur Monster

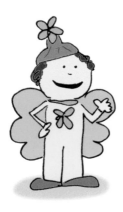

Flower

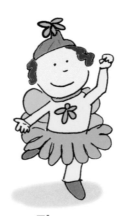

Flower Ballerina

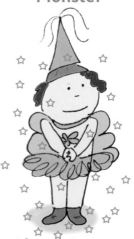

Glitter Princess Flower Ballerina

Play-by-Play
With Chuck and Judy

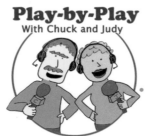

OPENING GIFTS

Toddler has received an impressive pile of holiday gifts, and Mom and Dad are excited to watch everything get opened. Let's get the play-by-play report from our commentators, Chuck and Judy, who are live on the scene.

Judy, it's go time! Toddler is ready to open the gifts!

Chuck, that's quite a pile of presents there. Look at that huge one!

I know! But Toddler seems focused on the smaller gift with the pretty bow.

She's going for that one!

Wow, I don't think I've ever seen anyone rip paper that fast.

It's like someone hit fast-forward.

That was a blur. But now she has the gift in hand!

It's a pack of three small princess figurines.

Price tag is still on. Looks like a $5.00 gift. Boy, she loves these little princesses.

Loves them!

She's sitting down, starting to play with them.
But wait . . . what are Mom and Dad saying?

They want her to keep opening gifts.

But she already found one she loves!

They're really pushing, Chuck.
They're handing her another present.

Whoa! She swatted it away. But wait . . .
she's picking up the bow that was on the gift.
She likes that bow. Very, very focused on the bow.

What about that huge present in the corner?

Judy, at this point, all the other gifts are just a nuisance.

You're right, Chuck. The gift opening is done
as far as Toddler is concerned.

It's time to leave her alone and let her play
with her favorite item: the bow.

Next: Chuck and Judy file a report at night-night time.

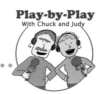

Holiday Helpers

Feel inferior when you read the holiday card about your neighbor's fabulous family? Just think of all the outstanding things *your* toddler accomplished this past year and you'll feel better.

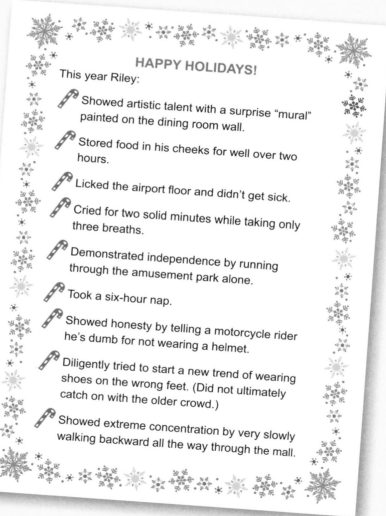

HAPPY HOLIDAYS!

This year Riley:

- Showed artistic talent with a surprise "mural" painted on the dining room wall.

- Stored food in his cheeks for well over two hours.

- Licked the airport floor and didn't get sick.

- Cried for two solid minutes while taking only three breaths.

- Demonstrated independence by running through the amusement park alone.

- Took a six-hour nap.

- Showed honesty by telling a motorcycle rider he's dumb for not wearing a helmet.

- Diligently tried to start a new trend of wearing shoes on the wrong feet. (Did not ultimately catch on with the older crowd.)

- Showed extreme concentration by very slowly walking backward all the way through the mall.

TODDLER HANDBOOK
TIPS FOR TODDLERS, BY TODDLERS

CHEESE!
If someone is trying to take your holiday picture, be sure to flash your "picture smile." Do not veer from this smile. Also, do not listen to anyone who tells you to "smile naturally." They have no clue what they're talking about.

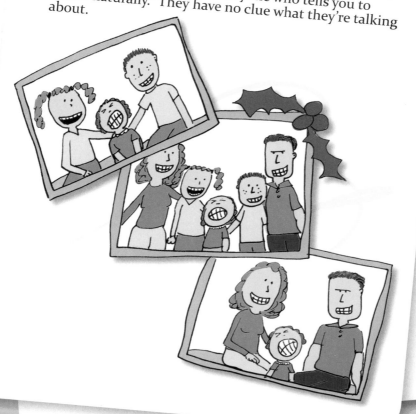

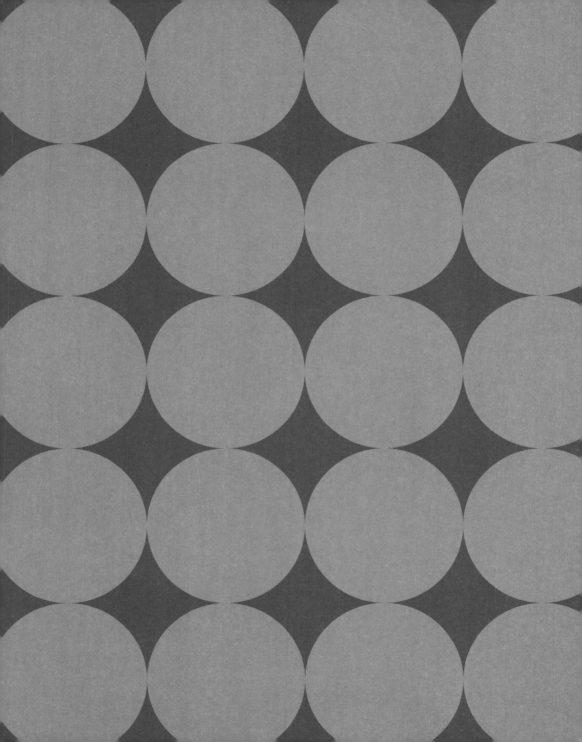

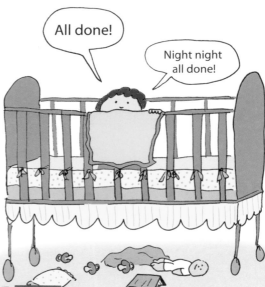

Chapter 8

NIGHT- NIGHT!

Sleep. It hasn't been easy since your darling child was born.

Sure, Toddler may be sleeping through the night most of the time. But probably not all nights. And now that Toddler can talk, he is coming up with stall tactics, urgent demands, and bizarre requests whenever it's time for bed. Then there are the routines that must be followed, the bedtime items that must be arranged just so, and the midnight visits to crowd you out of your bed.

It's exhausting just thinking about it. Are you exhausted? All right then. Snuggle up and let's talk about sleep.

SPOT THE TODDLER

Before they even think about falling asleep, toddlers insist on being surrounded by toys, blankets, pillows, stuffed animals, and more. Can you spot the toddler?

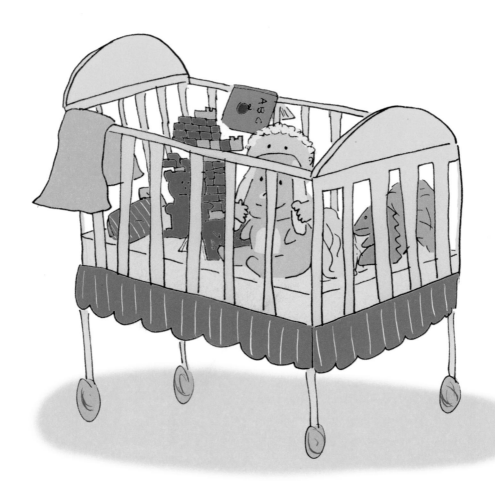

TIRED TODDLER MOOD RING

When a toddler gets overtired, there's no telling how she will react. Put a mood ring on her and use this guide to decipher the state of her emotions.

 Yellow: Chipper. Excited to read book.

 Orange: Edgy. Things like the sound of a parent texting can set toddler off.

 Pink: Extra hyper. Toddler can often be found frantically pulling books off of shelf while hooting like a howler monkey.

 Purple: Totally unbalanced mix of sadness and hyperactivity. May jump on couch while singing favorite song, then crumple in a heap when he can't remember all of the words.

 Brown: Angry. Upset with rules, naps, family, windows, sippies, stairs, soap, anything.

 Deep blue: Extremely emotional. It's as if Toddler just watched *Titanic* and *The Notebook* back to back.

 Light green: Catatonic. Staring straight ahead at nothing . . . blinks becoming slower.

 Light blue: Asleep at last.

LET THE FUN BEGIN!

Why do toddlers fuss so much at naptime? Because they are convinced that they are missing out on incredible fun. Let's take a look.

What Is Actually Happening During Nap Time	What Toddlers Think Is Happening
You are running all over picking up the house and doing laundry.	A parade of puppies and kittens is prancing and rolling through the living room, looking for a little kid to play with.
You are responding to e-mail and paying bills.	All of Toddler's friends have come over to drink chocolate milk, watch a cartoon, and take pony rides around the front yard.
You are returning phone calls.	A huge gumball machine has been wheeled into the kitchen and is dispensing gum and candy left and right. Little toys and juice boxes are also pouring out.

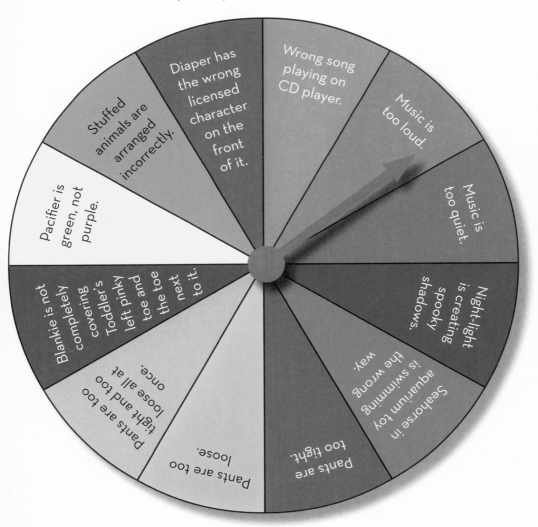

WHEEL OF UNACCEPTABILITY

What may upset Toddler during nap time? To find out, let's spin the wheel of unacceptability.

Wrong song playing on CD player.

Music is too loud.

Music is too quiet.

Night-light is creating spooky shadows.

Seahorse in aquarium toy is swimming the wrong way.

Pants are too tight.

Pants are too loose.

Pants are too tight and too loose all at once.

Blankie is not completely covering Toddler's left pinky toe and the toe next to it.

Pacifier is green, not purple.

Stuffed animals are arranged incorrectly.

Diaper has the wrong licensed character on the front of it.

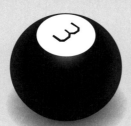

Ask the Magic 3 Ball

Ask the Magic 3 Ball and tap into a three-year-old's wisdom

Toddler: Instead of taking a nap, should I get the diaper cream and rub it all over my body?

Magic 3 Ball:

Yes and no.

Don't get the cream in your eyes, but do rub it on your cheeks, so that your parents fear you swallowed it and call Poison Control. That will buy you ten more minutes of awake time!

TODDLER HANDBOOK

TIPS FOR TODDLERS, BY TODDLERS

WHEN AND WHEN *NOT* TO WAKE UP FROM A NAP

Time to wake up! **Do not wake up.**

Your mom sits down and quietly cracks open a book.

Your older sibling just left for a playdate. The house is quiet and peaceful.

Sounds like Mom might be on an important conference call for work.

Your mom is vacuuming, unloading the dishwasher, and making a ton of noise in an attempt to rouse you from your slumber.

Your family is invited to a special event and you need to get dressed and ready right now.

It's errand day! There are lots of places that Mom needs to go.

THE BIG BED!

When is Toddler ready for a big bed? There are four signs:

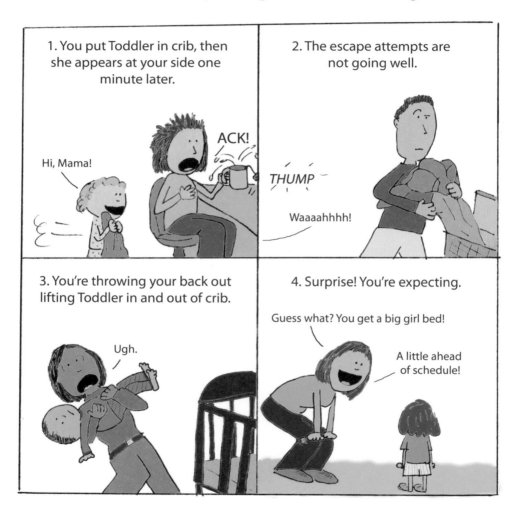

BEDTIME BINGO

Which behavior are you seeing today?

B	E	D	T	I	M	E
I'm thirsty!	I spilled my water!	I need socks!	I need a Band-Aid!	I need to go pee!
One more hug!	I don't want my socks on!	My closet is open!	My closet is still open a tiny crack!	I have to tell you something!
Where is my pillow?	I hear something!	Rub my back!	I need a snack!	I'm afraid of my clock!
My eyes are broken!	I can't fall asleep!	I need another book!	Are monsters real?!	How many hours till my birthday?
I don't like my crib!	When can I get up?	I dropped my toy!	I dropped my toy again!	Is it daytime yet?

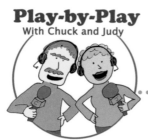

Play-by-Play
With Chuck and Judy

READING TIME

The day is ending for Toddler. Let's cut to our commentators, Chuck and Judy, who will give us a play-by-play report live from the scene.

Chuck, it looks like night-night time.

Yes.

Toddler is picking a book.

He seems to be deciding between that super short one and the really, really long one. Ah! He's going with the really, really long one.

Chuck, Toddler wants Dad to lie down next to him and read. But that toddler bed is pretty tiny.

Dad is contorting his body . . . bending . . . folding in on himself . . . tucking the leg . . . there! Whoa! I didn't think he could pull that off.

Toddler wants to hold the book.

Of course.

Dad is reading. Uh-oh, looks like he tried to skip a page!

Judy, that is not going to fly.

That's right, Chuck. Toddler has memorized every line of this book. If Dad so much as tries to skip one word, Toddler will know.

He better not turn those pages too fast, either. It takes Toddler a while to really examine and appreciate the art.

Naturally.

Well, Judy, it looks like these two are going to be at it for a long, long, long time. Let's wish them well and sign off.

Sweet dreams, Chuck.

Sweet dreams.

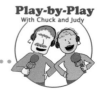

Play-by-Play
With Chuck and Judy

NOTES FOR THE BABYSITTER

From the Desk of Toddler's Mommy

Dear Katie,

Thank you for babysitting for us tonight. Here are some notes about putting Bobby to bed. Best of luck!

1. Bobby needs to be situated at a 30-degree angle to the door, with his yellow blanket (light yellow, not dark yellow) covering him just up to his chest, one-half centimeter lower than his armpits.

2. Placement of the stuffed animals: If you imagine an equilateral triangle, where Bobby's head is at the point A (top), you'll want to put his bunny at point B (left) with the face looking straight up at the ceiling. You'll want to put the bear at point C (right), and the bear should be looking at the bunny. Position the bunny first, then the bear. Do not attempt to do it the other way around.

From the Desk of Toddler's Mommy

3. Now sing the ABC song to him, in a British accent—specifically the type of accent you would find in the Northern Midlands of Britain (think Yorkshire). Do not morph into an Australian accent. Do not. Just trust us on that.

4. When ABC concludes, begin to sing "Twinkle Twinkle Little Star" (maintaining the Yorkshire accent) and then take a step back. Spin slowly (360 degrees) then take another step. Spin again and repeat until you are in the hall.

5. Continue singing "Twinkle Twinkle Little Star" until he falls asleep or until we get home.

Thank you! We'll be home very late.

NIGHTTIME CUTENESS

Toddlers may be a handful during the day, but they know one way to redeem themselves: by looking extra adorable at night.

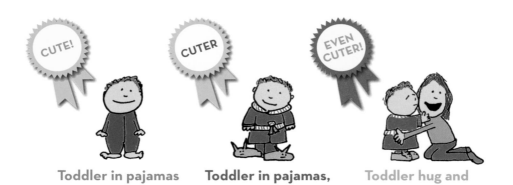

Toddler in pajamas   **Toddler in pajamas, robe, and slippers**   **Toddler hug and kiss goodnight**

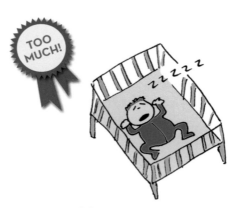

Toddler singing in crib   **Toddler sleeping in "bug" position from babyhood**

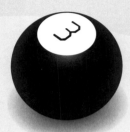

Ask the Magic 3 Ball

Ask the Magic 3 Ball and tap into a three-year-old's wisdom

Toddler: I don't want to sleep and I'm tired of crying it out. Should I throw up?

Magic 3 Ball:

It is decidedly so.

Crying takes too much energy; it's more effective and expedient to throw up. Chances are very good that "night-night time" will be "all done."

Toddler Handbook

Tips for Toddlers, by Toddlers

FAMILY SLUMBERING

- In the middle of the night, run down the hallway without bothering to tiptoe. Your parents will hear the pitter-patter of your feet and be grateful that you are coming to join them in bed at such an hour.

- Climb onto the bed, find a warm body, and lie directly on top of it, horizontally.

- You will likely be moved. There is no need for you to cooperate in this matter. Just let your entire body go limp as your parents try to reposition you.

- Once they position you, rotate yourself so you are horizontal again. Your feet should be pressing against the side of one parent's face and your hands should be flopping against your other parent's face.

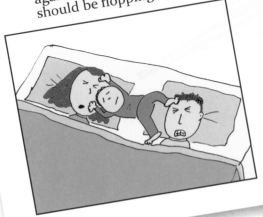

Correct position.

✏️ As you drift back to sleep, don't worry about disrupting anyone with your kicking, elbowing, snoring, or flopping around. None of this is your concern.

✏️ If you feel you must pee, then pee.

✏️ By the time everyone wakes up, you should be not only horizontal but also spread eagle with your arms stretched out above your head. Your parents should be pushed so far to the side that they are almost falling off the edge of the bed.

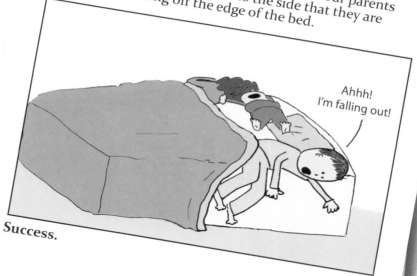

Success.

NIGHTMARE!

A quick look at what frightens toddlers versus what frightens adults.

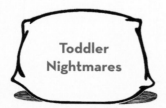

Toddler Nightmares

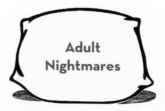

Adult Nightmares

Toddler Nightmares	Adult Nightmares
Being chased by a squirrel	Being chased by bill collectors
Tiny man wearing strange sweater	Tiny mouse in chest of sweaters
Battery running out in toy	Battery running out in cell phone
Oatmeal	Trying to feed Toddler oatmeal
Getting hair brushed	Losing hair
No one paying attention	Speaking in front of a large group
Not being able to run around naked	Running around naked
Being forced to wear a diaper	Being forced to wear a diaper

RISE AND SHINE

The lovely ways that toddlers wake their parents at 5:30 a.m.

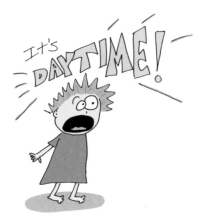

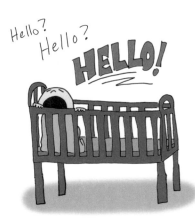

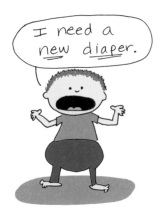

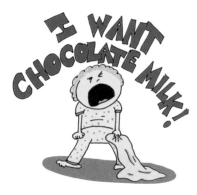

And another day begins
in The World According
to Toddlers . . .

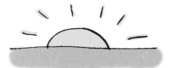

THE END?

The toddler years may be bizarre, but eventually they do draw to a close. Your pint-sized tyrant becomes less emotional. More reasonable. A better companion overall.

At last, you can congratulate yourself: You made it through a difficult period. It's smooth sailing now. All the irrational and dramatic behavior is behind you. The absurd demands, emotional outbursts, and crazy displays of willpower and negotiation—gone for good!

Well, wait a minute. Maybe not for good . . .

The World According to TEENS

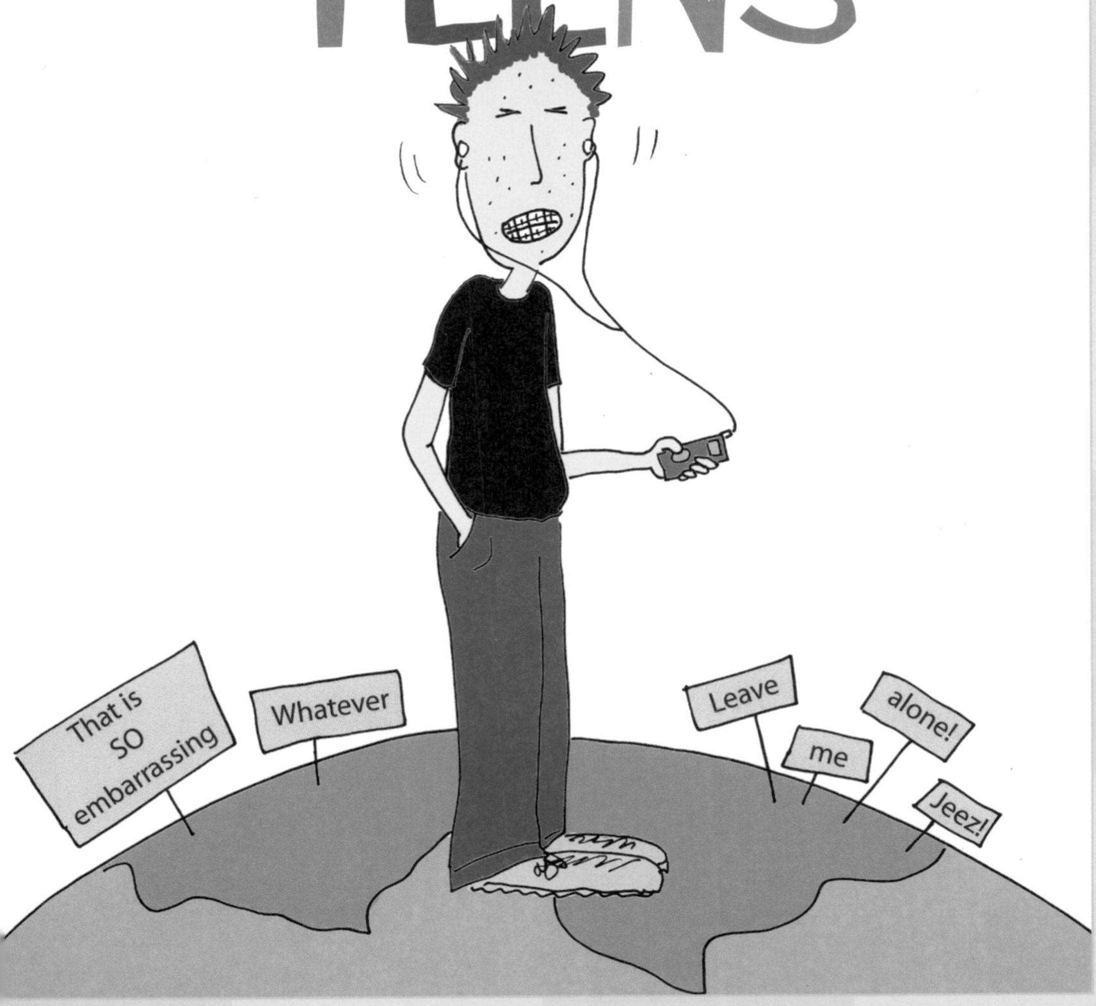

ADRIENNE HEDGER

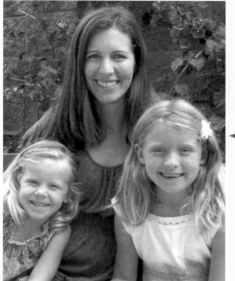

Photos by Krista Sinacori

Kate: Perfected the technique of launching a huge tantrum, suddenly pausing to carefully lie down on the floor, then resuming the tantrum full force.

Claire: Famous for always clutching a teetering pile of blankies, stuffed animals, dolls, shoes, and other treasured items so no one else could touch them.

**SHANNON
PAYETTE SEIP**

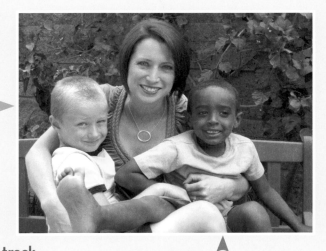

Isaac: Excelled at running off in crowded airports and bursting into tears if train derailed from toy track.

Bini: Shenanigans include sneaking out in Wisconsin winter and turning on garden hose— four months of streaming water led to $4,000 water bill.

A big thank-you to our friends, family members, and all the parents and grandparents who shared their toddler stories with us. Remember, we're all in this together. Find the humor!

We also want to thank our kids who, with their mind-boggling mischievousness, provided much material for this book.

The fun continues at

http://www.TheWorldAccordingToToddlers.com.

▶ Come check it out!